7.95

MIND AND VISION

MIND AND VISION

A HANDBOOK FOR THE CURE OF IMPERFECT
SIGHT WITHOUT GLASSES

DR. R. S. AGARWAL

SCHOOL FOR PERFECT EYESIGHT
SRI AUROBINDO ASHRAM
PONDICHERRY

First Edition: 1935
Reprinted: 1941, 1944, 1947, 1955
Revised Edition: 1972
Seventh Edition (Facsimile): 1978
Second Impression: 1983
Third Impression: 1986
Fourth Impression: 1990

ISBN 81-7058-218-O

Published by Sri Aurobindo Ashram, Publication Department
Printed at Sri Aurobindo Ashram Press, Pondicherry
PRINTED IN INDIA

CONTENTS

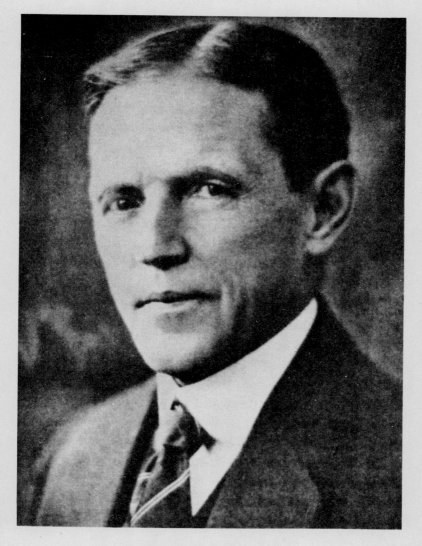

DR. W. H. BATES M. D.
Ophthalmologist and discoverer of the cure of imperfect
sight by treatment without glasses.

INTRODUCTION

Preservation of good eyesight is almost impossible without proper eye education and mental relaxation. The quieter the mind, better is the eyesight preserved.

It is a fact that glasses help many to relieve their discomforts of their head and eyes and enable people to see well at a distance or near, and their use in many cases is imperative. But this is also true that glasses do not check further deterioration and the number of glasses goes on increasing. Often glasses become an added torture to increase the pain and suffering and loss of eyesight. The fast deterioration in eyesight and the development of some serious complications are not prevented by the use of glasses, injections and pills. Therefore, the number of blind people amongst the educated class is fast increasing in spite of all possible medical aid.

The orthodox belief is that for cases of defective eyesight as myopia and hypermetropia and astigmatism, there is not only no cure, but practically no preventive also. Any rational mind will think such a claim as dogmatic, an imperfection in the ophthalmic science. When the sight begins to deteriorate, there must be some cause for it, and the cause is always an effort to see or strain. The eye being a sense organ is closely associated with the mind in its functioning, and like other sense organs makes no effort to see in its normal course. The normal eye when it makes an effort to see at a distance, its distant vision becomes defective and myopia is produced. When the normal eye makes an effort to see at a near point, its near vision becomes defective and hypermetropia is produced. Glasses neutralize the effect of such conditions but do not relieve the cause of the trouble. So, in many cases, the cause continues increasing by the use of glasses and the sight goes on deteriorating.

It is a well-known fact that vision is a process of mental interpretation. The picture which the mind sees is not the impression on the retina, but a mental interpretation of it. For example, to the good eye the white centre of letter O seems to be whiter than the margin of the page, this is because the mind interprets the retinal image in this way. Therefore, our vision mostly depends on our mind's imagination. When the imagination is perfect, sight is perfect. But if the imagination is imperfect, sight also is recorded imperfect.

The old writers on ophthalmology did not consider that the mental strain could play an important part in the formation of errors of refraction, hence they isolated the eye while determining the cause and treatment of visual defects and retinal disorders. To rectify the effect of errors of refraction they prescribed glasses. But very little has ever been claimed about their usefulness except that these contrivances neutralize the effects of the various conditions for which they are prescribed, as a crutch enables a lame man to walk. This incurability of errors of refraction is based on the theory that the eye changes its focus for vision at different distances by altering the curvature of the lens.

It struck to Dr. W. H. Bates M.D., an American Scientist, that further experiments and observations were necessary to determine the facts about accommodation and errors of refraction. His experiments are a proof that the lens is not a factor in accommodation. The eye adjusts its focus for different distances just like a camera, by a change in the length of the organ, and this alteration is brought about by the action of external eye muscles, called oblique muscles. Dr. Bates has made many remarkable discoveries regarding the refraction of the eye but the most remarkable discovery of Dr. Bates is: FINE PRINT IS A BENEFIT TO THE EYES WHILE LARGE PRINT IS A MENACE. The reason is that while reading fine print one sees a tiny area at a time, while in reading large print one has to see a large area at a time and the eye feels strain in such an attempt.

Dr. Bates' discoveries are a boon to humanity. Thousands of cases, so-called incurable, have been benefited by his simple methods of treatment. For example, a woman who had developed total night blindness was completely cured in about a month's time. And a boy who had become semi-blind, gained normal vision in a couple of weeks. A German lady who had developed squint by the wrong use of the eyes was cured in about two weeks time. Cases of incipient cataract, glaucoma, retinal disorders, floating specks, amblyopia, etc., have derived great benefit by the system of eye education.

All along it has been my experience that mental relaxation is the key to success in life, in education and treatment. Under the present conditions of life, man's mind is under a severe strain, hence preservation of good eyesight has become almost impossible without eye education. One may have good eyesight today but will not be able to preserve it after some time. If children and adults are taught about the proper use of the eyes, most of the visual defects will fade away in due course of time and man will enjoy perfect eyesight. Though glasses are also necessary in some cases, yet unless the prescription of glasses is supplemented by eye education deterioration in eyesight and blindness cannot be prevented.

For practical working in an efficient way a synthesis of all the systems of medicine is necessary. In this synthesis eye education will play an important part in the prevention and cure of most eye troubles. Here I give a few hints about eye education:

1. BLINKING: Blinking is a continuous habit of good eyes. By blinking the eyes work under rest, the habit of staring is checked. While reading one should blink at each line, while seeing some distant object shift the sight from part to part and blink.

2. PALMING: By palming I mean to close the eyes and cover them with the palms of hands in such a way that there is no pressure on the eye-balls and no light enters the eyes. Now a complete black field will be observed before the eyes. Palming when done in the right way, makes the mind quiet and gives good relaxation.

3. SUN TREATMENT: Facing the morning sun with eyes closed for a few minutes while moving the body gently from side to side like a pendulum, improves the health of the eyes and cures day blindness.

4. READING SNELLEN TEST CARD daily is very helpful to prevent and cure myopia and other visual defects in the schools.

5. READING FINE PRINT daily is extremely beneficial to the eyes.

BLIND NOTIONS: Reading fine print is commonly supposed to be harmful to the eyes, and reading print of any kind in dim light and close to the eyes is regarded as a dangerous practice. Due to such a belief a student suffered a lot. He had pain in the eyes and pain in the head, he was in a state of agony and lost his peace of the mind and his health was affected. When he began to read fine print in candle light and good light alternately at a close distance, surprisingly all his pain in the eyes was chased away in three days and was relieved from headache.

In the School for Perfect Eyesight we have evolved a system of practical working based on the synthesis of all the systems of medicine. We believe that all the methods of treatment as glasses, medicines, operation and eye education have their utility but the efficacy of eye education and mental relaxation is so great that often one can successfully treat cases of visual defects and eye troubles even without a diagnosis. The reason is that when a patient complains of pain, headache and loss of vision, it is an indication of eye strain and mental strain; and the treatment which will relieve the strain will be beneficial to the eyes. I may mention here about the discovery of a new technique called 'the art of seeing pictures and view-cards.' This technique when done perfectly brings quick cure in some cases of visual defects. Two girls had developed bad eyesight both for distance and near, a condition of semi-blindness (Amblyopia). Formerly such cases usually took about two weeks or more for the cure but by the art of seeing pictures they got cured in a few minutes. They were given a view-card of Taj Mahal Agra and were taught the art of seeing with the mind perfectly relaxed. When the flatness of the picture disappeared and the three-dimensional character of the picture was clearly perceived, the picture appeared so beautiful to the eyes of the girls that their minds got deeply absorbed in seeing the Taj. They observed that the fine details of the picture were sharply coming up and the vision was getting improved. Then when the eyesight was tested on the Snellen Eye Testing Chart, it was recorded normal in 15 minutes.

We aim to create a new type of doctors who will bring perfection in eyesight and in general capacities of the mind and the body. Intuition will be their guide. Their knowledge will be based on the synthesis. They will be more concerned with the health than with the pathology. To achieve this aim the School for Perfect Eyesight provides a course in Ophthalmic Science. And I admit this fact that it is by the Grace of the Divine Mother and Sri Aurobindo that it has been possible to write this book 'MIND AND VISION'. There was a strong inspiration to express my thoughts and experiences, and in a strange way the opportunities arose with all facilities to complete this work. Often, Sri Aurobindo encouraged me with His letters and inner guidance to promote the work and lift it to its summit. His words *'These methods are perfectly effective'* are a great hope to the humanity to recover their lost eyesight.

DR. R. S. AGARWAL

CHAPTER I

THE ORGAN OF SIGHT

The essential parts of the visual apparatus are the eye or eyeball, certain nerve cells in the hinder part of the large brain, and nerve fibres connecting the eye with these cells. Vibrations of the ether, which are known as light, produce images of the outside world on the sensitive memberane, or retina at the back of the eye, thus stimulating the ends of the optic nerve whence impulses pass back to the brain and cause the sensation of light.

The eye is contained in a bony cavity in front of the skull known as the orbit, and is thus largely protected from external violence. Moreover, as the orbit is a roomy space, the eye, which with its attached muscles, is embedded in soft, fatty tissues, is afforded a sufficiently free range of movements. In front of the eye are lids with their lashes, which can close and protect the eye, while in the outer part of the upper lid is the tear-gland, which helps to keep the surface of the eye moist.

The eye presents to view a circular clear transparent membrane known as the cornea and beyond this, the white of the eye. The latter represents the sclerotic coat, a dense tough membrane — sclerotic is seen through the conjunctiva — which, except for the corneal surface, covers the eyeball. This is almost spherical, but if the eye is examined from the side, it will be seen that the cornea projects from the sclerotic part, just as a convex watch glass would do, were it applied to the surface of a circular orange. The cornea has no blood-vessels traversing it, but is plentifully supplied with nerves and is very sensitive. Within the sclerotic coat is the choroid, and inside this, the retina. The former has a free supply of blood-vessels and many pigment cells; it extends forward to near the junction of the cornea with the sclerotic coat, where it forms a large number of folds known as the ciliary processes, and beyond these is continuous with the outer circumference of the curtain of the eye, which is called the iris.

The iris may have a brown, blue or almost a greenish tint in different people, and is perforated by a central, circular opening, the pupil which can vary in size. This is because the iris contains two sets of muscle fibres, some circling round it, which contract the pupil and others radiating outwards, which dilate it. The iris is covered behind by a layer of pigment cells, which prevents light passing otherwise than through the pupil.

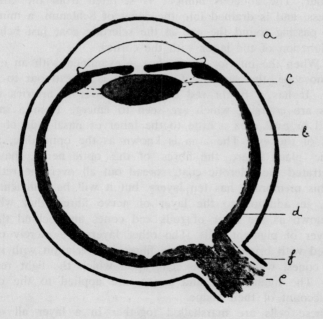

EYEBALL

a = Cornea	b = Sclera	c = Lens
d = Retina	e = Optic Nerve	f = Central Spot

Behind the iris is the crystalline lens of the eye which resembles a magnifying glass in miniature. It is enclosed in a capsule, and is supported all round its circumference by a membrane, the suspensory ligament of the lens, which, in turn, is attached to the ciliary processes.

If a section were made through an eyeball, it would be noted that the lens and the suspensory ligament divided the eye into a smaller front and a larger back portion. The former is further divided into what are called the anterior and the posterior chambers of the eye; these are filled with aqueous, or watery humour. The space behind the lens is occupied by a clear, transparent jelly, known as the vitreous humour. The aqueous humour is secreted from the ciliary process, and is drained into the canal of Schlemm, a minute tube passing round the eye in the sclerotic coat just behind the junction of the latter with the cornea.

When the interior of the eye is examined with an ophthalmoscope, the surface of the retina is spread out to the view. It has a bright red colour and over it arteries and veins are coursing which are seen to emerge from a small round or oval area a little to the inner or nasal side of the back of the eye. The area is known as the optic disc, and is the place where the fibres of the optic nerve, having penetrated the sclerotic coat, spread out all over the retina.

This membrane has ten layers, but it will be sufficient to note, in addition to the layer of nerve fibres, that which is known as the layer of rods and cones and behind these a layer of pigment cells. The other layers are merely concerned with bringing the nerve fibres into relation with rods and cones, which are the cells upon which the light really acts. The names rods and cones, are applied to the cells on account of their shape.

These cells are marshalled together in a layer all over the retina, except that there are none of them on the optic disc, and consequently there is no perception of light here. At the centre of the back of the eye, there is a little area which, from its colour, is called the macula lutea, or the yellow spot. At its centre, there is a little pit or depression, the fovea centralis, which represents the part of retina where visual perception is sharpest in ordinary illumination. It is noteworthy that lining this part, and close round it, there are only cones. On the outlying parts of the retina, however, where vision is the best in a subdued light, the rods form a great majority.

Each optic nerve passes backwards and enters the skull through an opening at the back of the orbit. Just after doing so, the fibres, which supply the inner or nasal portion of the retina cross to the other side, the band formed by these and other crossing fibres being known as the optic commissure or chiasma.

From the commissure, the fibres pass back in the optic tract on either side to flat projections on the base of the brain called the corpora quadrigemina, in the neighbourhood of which are nerve cells forming relay stations on the way to the back part of the brain and which also act as reflex centres for the movements of the pupil. Light, that is to say, falling on the retina, produces a nerve impulse which is carried to these cells, and an impulse comes back causing the pupil to contract.

From the relay stations fibres carry visual impressions to the back parts of the occipital lobes, of the brain, to nerve cells in the cortex, or the superficial part of the brain substance, where the sensation of light is appreciated; from these cells, what are called association fibres link up farther forward on the brain with other cells concerned with the storage of images and the other intellectual aspects of vision.

When the eye is fixed on an object, the image of the latter is formed about the centre of the retina, and it is upside down; it is the mind, therefore, which enables us to see things in their correct positions. If one eye is covered, besides seeing the particular object looked at, one sees more or less of its surroundings, and all that is visible is

called the field of vision of the eye. Although one is not
ordinarily aware of it, there is a small area which is not
seen. This corresponds to the optic disc, and lies outside
the object looked at. If right eye is closed and the gaze
of the left eye is fixed on the square shown here, the
page being held about 10 inches away, it will be noticed
that, as the page is brought near the eye, the round dot
disappears, but reappears when the page is brought still
nearer. It disappears because rays from it fall on the insen-
sitive optic disc. The area on the field of vision corresponding to the disc is called the blind spot.

Demonstration of Blind Spot

Ocular Muscles: — There are six muscles on the outside
of the eyeball, four known as the "recti" and two as the
"obliques". The obliques form an almost complete belt
round the middle of the eyeball, and are known, according
to their position, as "superior" and "inferior".

The "recti" are attached to the sclera or outer coat of
the eyeball near the front, and pass directly over the top,
bottom and sides of the globe to the back of the orbit,
where they are attached to the bone round the edges of the
hole through which the optic nerve passes. According to
their position, they are known as the "superior", "inferior",

"internal" and "external" recti. The obliques are the muscles of accommodation; and are concerned in the production of myopia; the recti are concerned in the production of hypermetropia and astigmatism.

THE EYE AS A CAMERA

The eye sees clearly at different distances — sometimes near and sometimes far. This power of changing the focus at different distances is brought about by the change in its length as in the camera.

The eye is compared with the camera in its structure, but the adjustment necessary for focussing the image of the object at different distances is said to be different. That is, in the camera the adjustment is affected by a change in the length of the body, but in the eye, according to Helmholtz, by a change in the lens and ciliary muscle. Dr. Bates' experiments on different animals and patients prove that the eye also, like the camera, adjusts its focus by a change in the length of the eyeball, this alteration being brought about by the action of the muscles on the outside of the eyeball and not by the lens and the ciliary muscle.

In one respect, however, there is a great difference between the two instruments. The sensitive plate of the camera is equally sensitive in every part; but the retina has a point of maximum sensitiveness, and every other part is less sensitive in proportion as it is removed from that point. This point of maximum sensitiveness is called the "fovea centralis", literally the central pit. This point is the seat of clearest vision. As we withdraw from this spot, the acuteness of visual perception rapidly decreases. The eye with normal sight, therefore, sees one part of everything it looks at best, and everything else worse, in proportion to the removal of the object from the point of maximum vision.

If we compare the picture on the glass screen of the camera when the camera is out of focus with the visual impressions of the mind when the eye is out of focus, there will be a great difference between them. When the camera is out of focus, it turns black into grey, and blurs the outlines of the picture; but it produces the results uniformly and constantly. On the screen of the camera, an imperfect picture of a black object would be equally imperfect in all parts, and the same adjustment of the focus would always produce the same picture. But when the eye is out of focus, the imperfect picture, which the patient sees, is always changing whether the focus changes or not. There will be more grey on one part than on the other. Again, the black may be changed into brown, yellow, green or even red, transmutations impossible to the camera.

When the camera is out of focus, the picture, which it produces, of any object is always slightly larger than the image produced when the forcus is correct; but when the eye is out of focus, the picture, which the mind sees, may be either larger or smaller than it normally would be.

When the human eye is out of focus, the form of the object regarded by the patient frequently appears to be distorted. The image may be doubled, tripled or still further multipled. The location of objects may also appear to change. Nothing like this could happen when the camera is out of focus.

These aberrations of vision are illusions, and not due to the fault of the eyes. It is because we see very largely with the mind and partly with the eyes. The phenomena of vision depend upon the mind's interpretation of the impression upon the retina. What we see is not that impression, but our own interpretation of it. The moon looks smaller at the zenith than it does at the horizon though the optical angle is the same and the impression on the retina may be the same, as at the horizon the mind unconsciously compares the picture with the pictures of the surrounding objects, while at the zenith, there is nothing to compare it with.

Therefore, the act of seeing is passive. Things are seen

just as they are felt, or heard, or tasted, without effort or volition on the part of the subject. No two persons with normal sight will get the same visual impressions from the same object; for their interpretations of the retinal picture will differ as much as their individualities differ. When the sight is imperfect, the interpretation is far more variable. Nothing like this happens in the case of two cameras.

In a camera, the blurred image is brought to focus by lengthening or shortening the body of the camera. When the image in the eye is out of focus, the eyesight is said to be defective and one consciously or unconsciously makes an effort to see objects and the mind goes out of control. The muscles of the eye, which lengthen or shorten the axis of the eyeball work under the control of the mind. When the mind is at rest, they work properly and the sight is normal. When the mind is under strain, they work imperfectly, and imperfect sight is the result. By the education of the mind and the eyes through some exercises, the muscles of the eye can be trained to bring the blurred image to a focus. (*See diagram on the next page.*)

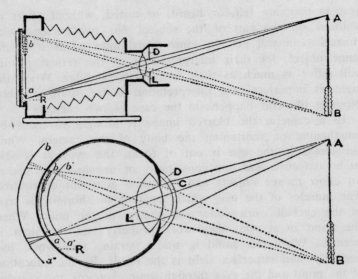

The Eye and Camera

OBJECT OF VISION AB — *Object to be photographed in the camera or the eye.*

ab — image on the sensitive plate or retina.

a'b' — image in the hypermetropic eye.

a"b" — image in the myopic eye.

DIAPHRAGM D — *In the camera, the diaphrcgm is made up of circular overlapping plates of metal by means of which the opening, through which the rays of light enter the chamber, can be enlarged or contracted.*

In the eye, the iris acts as a diaphragm and has a natural capacity for dilating and contracting the opening called the pupil of the eye.

LENS L. — *The lens behind the diaphragm, where the light rays are refracted.*

SENSITIVE PLATE R — *The sensitive plate in the camera or the retina of the eye, for receiving the image of the object.*

ACCOMMODATION

The power of the eye to change its focus for vision from distance to a near point is called accommodation. It is generally believed (a) that the lens of the eye under the control of the ciliary muscle regulates the vision by changing its convexity according to the distance of the object from the eye; (b) that the removal of the lens does away with the power of accommodation; (c) that the power of accommodation decreses from the age of forty and is completely lost after the age of sixty.

This theory about accommodation had been based on the images of Purkinji. If a small bright light, usually a candle, is held in front of and a little to one side of the eye, three images of the candle flame are seen:

1. Bright and upright — comes from the cornea, the transparent covering of the iris and pupil.
2. Large but less bright and upright — comes from the front of the lens.
3. Small, bright and inverted — comes from the back of the lens.

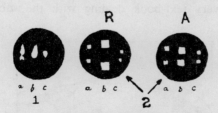

Images of Purkinji
a, on the cornea; b, on the front of the lens; c, on the back of the lens

Langenbeck examined these images with the naked eye and reached the conclusion that during accommodation the middle image coming from the front of the lens became smaller than what it was when the eye at rest was adjusted for distant vision. Since an image reflected from a convex surface is diminished in proportion to the convexity of that surface, he concluded that the front of the lens became more convex when the eye adjusted itself for near vision. Subsequently Helmholtz, working independently, made a similar observation, but by a somewhat different method. He found the image obtained by the ordinary methods on the front lens very unsatisfactory, and in his "Handbook of Physiological Optics," he describes it as being, "usually so blurred that the form of the flame cannot be definitely distinguished." so he placed two lights, or one doubled by reflection from a mirror, behind a screen in which were two small rectangular openings, the whole being so arranged that the lights shining through the openings of the screen formed two images on each of the reflecting surfaces. During accommodation, it seemed to him that the two images at the front of the lens became smaller and approached each other, while on the return of the eye to a state of rest, they grew larger again and separated. This change, he said, could be seen "easily and distinctly." The observations of Helmholtz regarding the behaviour of the lens in accommodation, published about the middle of the last century, were soon accepted as facts, and have ever since been stated as such in every text-book dealing with the subject.

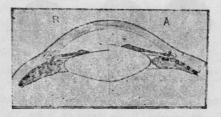

Diagram by which Helmholtz illustrated his theory of accommodation.

Dr. W. H. Bates, in the present century, repeated the experiments of Helmoltz in the Physiological Laboratory of the College of Physicians and Surgeons, Columbia University, New York, and New York City Aquarium. He was unable, however, by either of these methods, to obtain images that were sufficiently clear or distinct to be measured or photographed. With a thirty-watt lamp, a fifty-watt lamp, a 250-watt lamp and a 1,000-watt lamp, there was no improvement. The light of the sun, reflected from the front of the lens, produced an image just as cloudy and uncertain as the reflections from the other sources of illumination and just as variable in shape, intensity and size. To sum it all up, he was convinced that the anterior surface of the lens was a very poor reflector of light and that no reliable images could be obtained by the means described.

After many failures and hard work, Dr. Bates became able, with the aid of a strong light (1,000-watt), a diaphragm with a small opening and a condenser, to obtain photographs of images reflected from the front part of the lens both before and after accommodation. The images were clear and distinct; and, moreover, he arranged an apparatus by which an observer could see a clear image reflected from the cornea, the iris, the front part of the lens and the front part of the sclera. There was no change in the image reflected from the front part of the lens during accommodation at different distances. All his experiments in detail will be found in his book "Perfect Sight Without Glasses."

The corneal image was one of the easiest of the series to produce and the experiment is one which almost anyone can repeat, the only apparatus required being a fifty candle-power lamp — an ordinary electric globe — and a concave mirror fastened to a rod which moves back and forth in a groove so that the distance of mirror from the eye can be altered at will. A plane mirror might also be used; but the concave glass is better, because it magnifies the image. The mirror should be so arranged that it reflects the image of the electric filament on the cornea in such a way that the eye of a subject can see this reflection by looking straight ahead. The image in the mirror is used as the point of fixation, and the distance at which the eye focusses is altered by altering the distance of the mirror from the eye. The light can be placed within an inch or two of the eye, as the heat is not great enough to interfere with the experiment. The closer it is, the larger the image, and according to its being adjusted vertically, horizontally, or at an angle, the clearness of the reflection may vary. A blue glass screen can be used, if desired, to lessen the discomfort of light. If left eye is used by the subject — and in all experiments it was found to be more convenient for the purpose — the source of light should be placed to the left of that eye and as much as possible to the front of it, at an angle of about forty-five degrees. For absolute accuracy, the light and the head of the subject should be held immovable, but for demonstration, it is not essential. Simply holding the bulb in his hand the subject can demonstrate that the image changes according to the eye being at rest, accommodating normally for near vision, or, straining to see at a near or a distant point.

The image photographed from the cornea showed, however, a series of four well-marked changes, according to the vision being normal or accompanied by a strain. During accommodation the images from the cornea were smaller than when the eye was at rest, indicating elongation of the eyeball and a consequent increase in the convexity of the cornea. But when an unsuccessful effort was made to see at the near point, the image became larger, indicating that the cornea had become less convex, a condition which one would expect when the optic axis was shortened, as in hypermetropia. When a strain was made to see at a distance, the image was smaller than when the eye was at rest, again indicating elongation of the eyeball and increased convexity of the cornea, as in myopia.

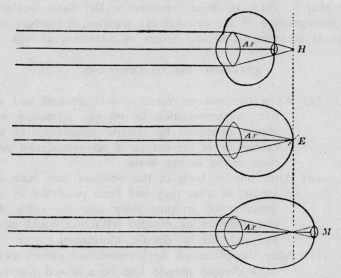

H, Hypermetropia; E, Normal; M, Myopia

SUMMARY

These studies of the images reflected from the various parts of the eyeball demonstrate that:

1. The accommodation of the eye is affected by an elongation of the eyeball.

2. The lens is not a factor in accommodation.

3. Myopia is produced by a strain to see distant objects.

4. Hypermetropia is produced by a strain to see near objects.

With these results, Dr. Bates reached the conclusion that the eye changes its focus by a change in its length, brought about by the action of the muscles on the outside of the eyeball.

To prove his own theory, Dr. Bates made many thousands of experiments on animals of all kinds, full details of which may be found in the New York Medical Journal for May 8, 1915. In these experiments, Dr. Bates was able by manipulation of the external eye muscles, to produce and prevent accommodation and errors of refraction at will.

EXPERIMENTAL OBSERVATIONS

1. (a) When two oblique muscles were present and active, accommodation or myopic refraction was always produced by electric stimulation of the eyeball or of the nerves of accommodation near their origin in the brain.

   (b) After one or both of the obliques had been cut across, or after they had been paralysed by the injection of atropine deep into the orbit, accommodation or myopic refraction could never be produced by electric stimulation.

   (c) After the effects of the atropine had passed away, or a divided muscle had been sewed together, accommodation followed electrical stimulation as before.

2. (a) If one or both of the oblique muscles had been cut, and two or more of the recti were present and active, electrical stimulation of the eyeball or of the nerves of accommodation, always produced hypermetropia.

   (b) The paralysing of the recti by atropine or, cutting of them, prevented the production of hypermetropia by electrical stimulation.

   (c) After the effects of the atropine had passed away or the divided muscles had been sewed together, hypermetropia was produced as usual.

3. Astigmatism was usually produced in combination with myopic or hypermetropic refraction. It was also produced by various manipulations of both the oblique and recti muscles. Mixed astigmatism, which is a combination of myopic with hyperme-

tropic refraction, was always produced by traction on the insertion of the superior or inferior rectus in a direction parallel to the plane of the iris, so long as both obliques were present and active; but if either or both of the obliques had been cut, the myopic part of the astigmatism disappeared. Similarly after the superior or the inferior rectus had been cut the hypermetropic part of the astigmatism disappeared. Advancement of the two obliques, with advancement of the superior and inferior recti, always produced mixed astigmatism.

4. Experiments performed on the lensless eye also showed the same results.

5. In the text-books on physiology of the eye, it is stated that accommodation is controlled by the third nerve, but experiments show that third and fourth nerves are equally important in accommodation.

(a) When either nerve is stimulated at the point of origin in the brain, accommodation or myopic refraction is always produced in the normal eye. When the origin is covered with a small pad of cotton soaked in a 2 per cent. atropine solution, stimulation of that nerve produces no accommodation, while stimulation of the unparalysed nerve produces it.

(b) When the action of the oblique muscles is prevented by dividing them, stimulation of the third nerve produces no accommodation but hypermetropia.

SUMMARY

Experiments on animals demonstrate that:

1. Neither the lens nor any muscle inside the eyeball has

anything to do with accommodation, but the process is entirely controlled by the action of the muscles on the outside of the eyeball.

2. Myopic refraction is always produced by a strain of two obliques and is always prevented by relaxation of these muscles by tenotomy (cutting).

3. Hypermetropic refraction is always produced by a strain of two or more recti, and is always prevented by relaxation of these muscles by tenotomy.

4. Astigmatism is produced by unsymmetrical changes.

5. Atropine prevents, when injected deep into the orbit, the experimental production of errors of refraction.

6. All errors of refraction are caused by strain in the muscles. The cure is accomplished by relaxation.

CLINICAL OBSERVATIONS

1. Many persons suffering from errors of refraction often recover their vision spontaneously. Errors of refraction disappear or change in their degree, after having been carefully diagnosed under atropine. Every ophthalmologist must have noted such cases. Different doctors often prescribe glasses of different powers to the same patient. If the eyeball is more or less a fixed organ and the error of refraction is a permanent one, then why should such differences occur?

2. In the case of disappearance or lessening of hypermetropia, we are asked to believe that the eye increases the curvature of the lens sufficiently to compensate for the flatness of the eyeball, both at the near point and at the distance. In the case of disappearance or lessening of myopia, ciliary muscle is credited with a capacity for getting into a more or less continuous state of contraction, thus keeping the lens continuously in a state of convexity. According to the theory, the lens can increase its convexity only for vision at the near point and not for distance.

3. It is believed that the lens changes its shape in moderate degrees of errors of refraction, and that only during the early years of life. For the variations of higher degrees, or those occuring after forty-five years of age, when the lens is supposed to have lost its elasticity to a greater or less degree, no plausible explanation has ever been devised.

4. If children are born with short or long eyes, then, why do they improve by Bates' methods?

5. If people who have had their lenses removed through a cataract operation follow Bates' methods, they can read fine print only with their distant glasses on at thirteen inches or even a less distance. Every ophthalmologist must have noted that only a minority of such cases can do the reading work very well with the distant glasses on.

In 1869 and 1870, respectively, Loring reported to the New York Ophthalmological Society and the American Ophthalmological Society "the case of a young woman of eighteen who, without any change in her glasses, read twenty feet line on the Snellen test card at twenty feet and also read fine print at a distance of five to twenty inches."

On October 8, 1894, a patient of Dr. A. E. Davis appeared to accommodate perfectly without a lens and consented to go before the New York Ophthalmological Society. "The members", Dr. Davis reported, "were divided in their opinion as to how the patient was able to accommodate for the near point with his distant glasses on."

These facts are offered as evidence that the lens is not a factor in accommodation, because the eye can change its focus within wide limits after the lens has been removed.

6. Astigmatism is said to be a permanent condition of the eye, but the disappearance of astigmatism, or changes in its character and axis present an even more baffling problem. Astigmatism can be produced voluntarily and some persons can produce as much as three diopters.

7. The cure of Presbyopia must also be added to the clinical testimony against the accepted theory of accom-

modation. In most of the cases, it can be easily demonstrated within a few minutes that the patient can read the finest print without glasses at a distance of 6 to 12 inches. On the theory that the lens is a factor in accommodation, such cures would be manifestly impossible when the lens is as hard as stone in old age.

The new theory is strengthened by accumulation of facts. The accepted theories of accommodation and of the cause of errors of refraction do not accord with facts and multitude of them have to be explained away. During more than thirty years of clinical experience, Dr. Bates did not observe a single fact that was not in harmony with his view that the lens and the ciliary muscle have nothing to do with accommodation, and that the changes in the shape of the eyeball, upon which errors of refraction depend, are not permanent. Clinical observations are also sufficient to show how errors of refraction can be produced at will, how they may be cured, temporarily, in a few minutes, and permanently by continued treatment.

CHAPTER II

EXAMINATION OF THE EYE

For practical work, specially when one has to deal with a large number of patients, it is not necessary to have a detailed examination of the eye. Two to ten minutes are quite sufficient for diagnosing the disease and prescribing the treatment. Even if it is difficult to diagnose a particular case or if it takes a long time, treatment can be begun safely. Use of atropine or other medicines which dilate the pupil are quite unnecessary in most cases as they often increase the strain in the eyes, specially in old age, and the examination of the eyes can be conveniently performed without their use. Some patients actually become blind by the use of atropine and we often see reports of such cases; but this fact is generally ignored and as a routine the eyes are examined under atropine or other medicines. Anyone who understands the application of the methods written in this book can successfully treat a case even if the diagnosis is not made. Some cases need prompt help and if much time is wasted in diagnosing such cases, all hope of recovery may be lost. Here we do not propose to give in detail the methods of eye-examination; if one feels interested one can study the subject from such books as 'Diseases of the Eye' by May and Worth.

When a patient presents himself for treatment, a record of his name, age and address is to be made. Then hear patiently the history and complaints of the patient and if necessary, have a few cross questions. The next procedure is to test the distant vision on the Snellen test card without and with glasses. Then the near sight is tested on the reading test type without and with glasses. Such records of eyesight are to be made from time to time during the course of the treatment. They give information of the improvement achieved. In some cases the improvement is so unconscious that the patient feels no improvement unless the records of vision are compared before him. The eyes are then examined with the ophthalmoscope or retinoscope. (The ophthalmoscope is valuable in diagnosing cataract, opacities of the cornea and diseases of interior of the eyeball. The retinoscope is used in diagnosing near-sightedness, far-sightedness and astigmatism.)

TEST OF DISTANT VISION

Place the Snellen Eye Testing Chart at 20 feet (6 metres) distance in good light at the level of the eyes. Read the chart with each eye separately, one eye being covered with the palm of the hand avoiding any pressure upon the eyeball. The vision is expressed by a fraction, the numerator of which corresponds to the number of feet separating the patient from the chart; and the denominator to the number written on the line read. If the sight is normal, the vision will be equal to 20 by 20 or 6 by 6. This is expressed D.V. (distant vision) 20 by 20. If one reads the first letter of the chart with the right eye and the third line with the left eye, then write R. E. (right eye)=20 by 200; L. E. (left eye)=20 by 70.

If no letter is seen at 20 feet, reduce the distance to 10 feet or 5 feet or 1 foot. Suppose the first letter is read at 5 feet, then write D. V. 5 by 200.

If you want to convert the figures in metres, divide the feet figures by ten and multiply by three, for example, 200 feet written on the top letter, 200/10x3=60 metres.

Another and even better way to test the sight is to compare the blackness of the letter of the Snellen eye chart at the near point and at twenty feet distance, in a dim light and in a good one. With perfect sight, black is not altered by illumination or distance. It appears just as black at the distance as at the near point, and just as black in a dim light as in a good one. If it does not appear equally black to you under all these conditions, therefore, you may know that your sight is imperfect.

TEST OF NEAR VISION

Generally two kinds of reading test types are used for testing near vision — one, Snellen test types, and the other, Jaegar's test types. The Fundamental test type-card is usually used for our work. Hold the test type at 12 inches, 9 inches and 6 inches or nearer. Read it with each eye covering the other eye with the palm of the hand or an eye-shield. The vision is expressed by F followed by the number corresponding to the finest print which one can read. Suppose No. 4 of F. Test type is read at 9 inches with the right eye, thus write R. E.=F4. at 9 inches.

NORMAL EYE

1. An eye with a perfect normal sight is rare; but for practical work a standard has been fixed. When the sight is normal for distance one reads the twenty feet line on the Snellen test card at twenty feet distance, and it is recorded as 20/20. When the sight is normal for near work, one reads the fine print at 9 to 12 inches.

2. The normal eye sees a small letter of the test card to be of the same size at 20 feet as it does at one foot. The white centres of the letters on the test card are imagined to be whiter than other parts of the card.

3. When the sight is perfect the letters on the test card seem to be perfectly black and perfectly distinct. The eye never tries to see them. The eye does not suffer from pain, discomfort or fatigue. The person is unconscious of his eyes.

4. When the normal eye regards a particular letter on the test card, the letter is seen better and blacker than all

the rest, and it seems as if the letter makes a slow, short and easy swing.

5. When a person with normal sight closes the eyes and covers them with the palms of his hands avoiding any pressure upon the eyeballs, he experiences a perfect black before the eyes as if he is in a perfectly dark room. This is because the retina of the eye reacts only to light and when there is no light it stops its function and one sees all perfectly black.

SEVEN TRUTHS OF NORMAL SIGHT

1. *Favourable conditions:* — Normal sight in the normal eye is present only under favourable conditions. Some people see in a bright light while others see better in a dim light. The distance at which the vision is at its best is widely variable. Some people may have normal vision at twenty feet but not at fifteen feet. Others are able to read fine print better at twelve inches than at six inches. By practice one can improve the vision so that it will be normal under all conditions.

When the eye regards an unfamiliar object, imperfect sight is always produced. Hence the proverbial fatigue caused by viewing pictures, or other objects, in a museum. A sudden exposure to strong light or rapid or sudden changes of light, are likely to produce imperfect sight in the normal eye. Under noise, unfamiliar sounds, mental and physical discomforts, errors of refraction are always produced in the normal eye. During sleep the eye is rarely normal, that is why people wake up in the morning with eyes more tired than at any other time, or even with severe headaches.

2. *Central Fixation:* — When the eye with the normal sight looks at a letter on the Snellen test card, it sees the letter regarded best, and all the other letters in the field of vision appear less distinct; this is called Central Fixation. As a matter of fact the whole letter and all the letters may

be perfectly black and distinct, and the impression that one
letter is blacker than the others or that one part of a letter is blacker than the others or that one part of a letter is
blacker than the rest, is an illusion.

3. *Shifting:* — The normal eye shifts rapidly from point
to point of a letter or an object, but the shifting is usually
not conspicuous. It is impossible for the eye to fix on a
point longer than a fraction of a second. If it tries to do
so, it begins to strain and the vision is lowered. This can
readily be demonstrated by trying to hold one part of a
letter for an appreciable length of time. No matter how
good the sight, it will begin to blur or even disappear very
quickly, and sometimes the effort to hold it will produce
pain.

4. *Swinging:* — When the eye with normal vision regards
a letter either at the near point or at the distance, the letter may appear to pulsate, or to move in various directions,
from side to side, up and down or obliquely. When it
looks from one letter to another on the Snellen test card,
or from one side of a letter to another, not only the letters but the whole line of letters and the whole card, may
appear to move from side to side. This apparent movement
is called swinging and is due to the shifting of the eye, and
is always in a direction contrary to its movement. While
riding in a fast moving train, the telegraph pole, although
fastened to the ground, appears to move in the opposite
direction.

5. *Perfect Memory:* — When the mind is able to remember perfectly the colour and the background of a letter, the
memory of the letter is instantaneous and continuous. If a
few seconds or longer are necessary to obtain the memory,
it is never perfect. When the memory is perfect the mind
is always perfectly relaxed, the sight is normal, if the eyes
are open; and when they are closed and covered so as to
exclude all the light, one sees a perfectly black field.

6. *Good Imagination:* — What we see through the eyes is

simply mind's interpretation of the retinal image. We see only what we think we see or what we imagine. When the imagination is perfect, the white part of the letters seems to be whiter than it really is, while black is not altered by distance, illumination, size, or form of the letters. For example, look at the white centre of the letter 'O' and compare the whiteness of the centre of 'O' with the whiteness of the rest of the card. The whiter you can imagine the centre of 'O' the better becomes the vision for the letter 'O'. The perfect imagination of the white centre of 'O' means perfect imagination of the black, because you cannot imagine the white perfectly, without imagining the black perfectly. (When the black is imagined perfectly it does not alter its shade by distance, illumination, size or form of the letters.)

7. *Rest:* — Rest or relaxation of the nerves of the eyes and mind is necessary before perfect vision can be obtained. When the eyes and mind are at rest, it is possible to remember, imagine or see all letters or other objects perfectly. It is not possible to remember, imagine, or see anything without perfect relaxation. Perfect rest or relaxation comes without effort. When the eye is at rest it is perfectly passive but never stationary; it is always moving.

When the sight is imperfect, these facts are not observed or are observed partly. If somehow they can be produced in the defective eye, the sight would become normal. This suggests the cure, and all exercises for the improvement of defective eyesight are based on these fundamental principles. It is impossible to observe these facts perfectly and at the same time to have defective eyesight. When one of these fundamental principles is perfect all others are perfect and the sight is also perfect. If one is able to observe them perfectly at three feet, the sight is normal at three feet; and if one is able to note at 20 feet, the sight is normal at twenty feet and so on.

CHAPTER III

GLASSES

It is true that the eye glasses have brought to some people improved vision and relief from pain and discomfort, but they do more or less harm to others. Glasses are nothing more than a very unsatisfactory substitute for normal vision.

It is a general belief that once the eye becomes defective, there exists no means whereby the eye can be brought to its normal condition; and for this, the spectacles were introduced. Having furnished the patient with suitable glasses, the eye specialist considers that he has done everything that lies within his power to cope with the abnormal condition; but it is a fact that the defect is not cured, it remains there and the sufferer is put only in a state of false satisfaction. The sufferer imagines that if he can see better, then his eyes must be better, and it is only after wearing spectacles for years, and having changed them more and more frequently for stronger ones, that the truth is borne in upon him that, instead of improving his eyes, the constant wearing of spectacles has made, in fact, the eyes worse, and will continue to do so.

It is true that all patients cannot attain normal vision due to imperfect practices and other circumstances. Therefore, to see clearly either for the distance or the near point, the patient requires glasses. If the oculist, while prescribing glasses, directs the patient to keep up blinking and practise Central Fixation for a few minutes every day, there would be no further deterioration of eyesight.

Prescription of glasses has increased so much that they are put on small children, and for little complaints. In some cases, though the vision is quite good, they are prescribed simply with the idea that there would be no deterioration of eyesight. Even if the patient resists the use of glasses, he is advised that if he would begin to use spectacles, there would be no further deterioration; otherwise the eyesight would go worse. The innocent patient is compelled to use them by such suggestions. After some time he finds the truth that the doctor gave him wrong advice, his eyesight is deteriorating. The wrong prescription of glasses causes harm to the eyes so much so that the eyes get very weak.

Many patients can be much benefited by the methods of relaxation, but if the glasses are to be prescribed, they should be of lowest possible power, and their use should be limited, that is, myopic patients may use for the distance and hypermetropic patients for the near. Constant use of glasses is harmful. When the patient complains of headache, the oculist tries to fit on glasses. Prescription of glasses in such cases often does not relieve headache. When the headache is not relieved, the patient runs from one doctor to the other and collects a number of spectacles. The cause of the headache is not defective sight but mental strain and improper use of the eyes. There are many who having very defective sight, use no glasses, work for long hours and still do not suffer from headache. There are others who have very good eyes, but often get headache. A doctor patient, who suffered from pain in the eyeballs while reading, was fitted with spectacles fifteen times by the specialists. He was relieved of the pain in a few minutes by the method prescribed in this book.

IMPORTANT POINTS

1. Glasses for the correction of far-sightedness (Hypermetropia) may, and usually do, give the wearer the impression that objects are larger than they really are; while near-sighted patients, when wearing glasses, are impressed with the fact that objects look smaller than they actually are.

2. In wearing the glasses, it is necessary to look directly through the centre of the glasses in order to obtain maximum

vision. If one regards an object by looking in a slanting direction through the glasses, its form and location are changed.

3. The discomfort from wearing the glasses is very great with a large percentage of people who use them. Frequently, when they complain to their doctors about the discomfort in wearing specially a new set of glasses prescribed, they are advised that by perseverance their eyes will become fitted to the glasses. This does not seem quite satisfactory, because the people feel that the glasses should fit their eyes, and not that they should struggle along with all kinds of discomfort in order to make their eyes fit the glasses.

4. Tinted glasses, red, yellow, blue, green or black, when worn constantly, are usually felt comfortable by the patient, because the amount of light is lessened. Constant wearing of such glasses is later followed by sensitiveness to light and the necessity of stronger glasses to obtain sufficient amount of relief. Constant protection of the eyes by dark glasses, shades and other measures often causes inflammation of the eyeball and of the eyelids, and poverty of vision.

5. Bifocal glasses sometimes cause discomfort to the eyes. The upper glass is meant to see distant objects, while the lower glass is meant for reading. One is not able to see through the junction between the two glasses. Hence one has to raise the eyeball to see distant objects and lower the eyeball to see the near objects. The eye is forced to move up and down in an unnatural way. This unnatural movement causes great strain on the eyes.

CHAPTER IV

THE CAUSE AND CURE OF ERRORS OF REFRACTION

How Does the Eye See?

The phenomena of seeing may be summarized as a result of three distinct processes:

1. *Mechanical*—the focussing action of the eye whereby the light rays in the form of an image are focussed on the sensitive film (the retina).

2. *Nervous*—the sensitivity of the retina in receiving the light rays and transmitting them to the visual centre in the brain.

3. *Mental*—the interpretation of the picture. Vision is a process of mental interpretation. The picture, which the mind sees, is not the impression on the retina, but a mental interpretation of it. The act of seeing is a passive one, and one sees involuntarily as one hears or tastes or smells.

The description of the normal eye with normal sight indicates that normal function of the eye is effortless, free from strain. While regarding an object or a letter it shifts rapidly from point to point and notes each part of the object regarded clearer than other parts. It has the normal refraction and normal sight only under favourable conditions which keep the eye and mind at rest. The unfavourable conditions cause strain on the eye and mind and imperfect sight is the result.

CAUSE OF ERRORS

If the strain on the mind due to unfavourable conditions persists and the eye consciously or unconsciously makes an effort to see, imperfect sight or an error of refraction is produced. More lasting habit of staring causes more lasting defect in eyesight.

When the eye makes an effort to see, it tries to see most of the part of an object at a time and does not shift rapidly from one point to another; it loses central fixation in this way and the vision gets blurred. For example, look at the notch at the top of the big 'C' of the Snellen test card at fifteen feet. Keep your eyes fixed on the notch without closing and shifting the eyes to some other point. Make an effort to see it and increase that effort as much as you possibly can. Notice that it is difficult to keep your eyes and mind fixed on that one point. Notice also that it is tiresome and it causes pain in the eyes. If you continue it long enough, your head begins to ache. If you look at some of the letters on the lower lines which are much smaller than the big 'C' they may appear so blurred that you are not able to distinguish them. Trying to see these small letters a little more blurs them still more.

Similarly fix the sight on a small letter at the reading distance and note that the letter is blurred.

EFFECT OF STRAIN

When one strains to see at a distance, the oblique muscles contract and lengthen the eyeball, the image of an object falls in front of the retina, and myopia or shortsightedness is produced; the focus of the eye is adjusted at a shorter distance, thus the distant sight becomes blurred. When the eye makes an effort to see at a near point the recti muscles contract and flatten the eyeball, the image of an object falls behind the retina, and hypermetropia or far-sightendness is produced; the focus is adjusted at a longer distance and not at a near point of reading, thus the near vision becomes blurred. When there is irregularity in action of the muscles, astigmatism is produced along with myopia or hypermetropia. When the eye suffers from myopia or hypermetropia or astigmatism, it is said that the eye has an error of refraction.

When a person with myopia strains at a distance, the degree of myopia is increased; and when he strains to see at a near point the myopia is lessened or disappears or even may become hypermetropic at that moment. If the hypermetropic eye strains to see a distant object, the hypermetropia is lessened and the vision improves. In some cases the hypermetropia is completely relieved. This condition may then pass over into myopia with an increase of strain. When the hypermetropic eye strains at a near point, hypermetropia is increased and the vision for reading becomes more blurred.

These facts explain that the eyes and mind are closely connected. The strain to see is a strain of the mind, and when there is a strain of the mind, there is a loss of mental control. Under the conditions of civilized life, men's minds are under a continual strain. They have more things to worry them than uncivilized men had, and they are not obliged to keep cool and collected in order that they may see and do other things upon which existence depends. If he allowed himself to get nervous, primitive man was promptly eliminated; but civilized man survives and transmits his mental characteristics to posterity.

The following conditions may cause the tendency to strain to see or increase the strain if it already exists:

1. By wrong use of the eyelids, that is by raising the upper lids and by stopping their gentle movement called blinking.
2. By using the eyes in a wrong way while reading, writing, sewing, seeing cinema, etc.
3. By moving the eyeballs in the opposite direction of the head and body, for example, if the head moves to the right and the eye to the left; or if the chin is downwards and the eyes look upwards. Physical eye exercises of rolling the eyeballs in various directions while keeping the head steady, as explained in various

books, are wrong and lead one to stare and increase the strain. The eye is purely a sense oragn and one cannot improve it by such physical exercises. All such efforts defeat the end in view.

4. By making an effort to see an object clearly, and by staring. Many people are unable to stare for any length of time; because staring is painful, disagreeable and produces fatigue. A boy, fourteen years of age, had practised staring and had acquired much skill in it; he was able to outstare any boy in his class-room. He then went to other classes and challenged each boy in those classes to a contest with him in staring. After sometime his eyes became inflamed and his vision became poor. Persons who stare at a dot or some other object without closing or shifting the eyes to practise *Yoga* usually suffer from myopia after sometime. A Swami practised staring and became highly myopic after sometime. It is a great mistake to think that staring at an object improves the mind or the sight.

5. By looking at unfamiliar objects, and by reading or seeing uninteresting and unpleasant things.

6. By going to the market or parties and trying to see there many things at a time.

7. By imitating those who have defective eyesight or those who strain while talking etc.

8. By fear, anxieties, worries, physical discomforts.

9. By imperfect imagination and distorted thoughts.

10. By excess of sexual appetite.

11. By using glasses unnecessarily.

12. By imagining unfamiliar and fearful dreams during sleep.

13. By exposing the eyes to strong heat; dust and smoke.

14. By using the eyes at the time when they require rest.

15. By insufficient nourishment.

VOLUNTARY PRODUCTION OF EYE TENSION, A SAFEGUARD AGAINST GLAUCOMA

It is a good thing to know to increase the tension of the eyeball voluntarily, as this enables one to avoid not only the strain that produces glaucoma; but other kinds of strain also. To do this proceed as follows:

Put the fingers on the upper part of the eyeball while looking downward, and note its softness. Then do any one of the following things:

(a) Try to see a letter or other object imperfectly, or (with the eye either closed or open) to imagine it imperfectly.

(b) Try to see a letter or a number of letters, all alike at one time, or to imagine them in this way.

(c) Try to imagine that a letter or mental picture of a letter is stationary.

(d) Try to see a letter or other object double or to imagine it double.

When successful, the eyeball will become harder in proportion to the degree of strain, but as it is very difficult to see, imagine, or remember things imperfectly, all may not be able at first to demonstrate the facts.

TREATMENT

The treatment of errors of refraction is not to avoid either near work or distant vision, but to get rid of the mental strain which underlies the imperfect functioning of the eye at both points. In all uncomplicated cases of errors of refraction the strain to see can be relieved, temporarily, by having the patient look at a blank wall without trying to see. To secure permanent relaxation sometimes requires considerable time and much ingenuity. The same method cannot be used with every one. The ways in which people strain to see are infinite, all the methods used to relieve the strain must be almost equally varied. Whatever the method that brings most relief, however, the end is always the same, namely relaxation or absence of an effort to see. By constant repetition and frequent demonstration, the fact must be impressed upon the patient that perfect sight can be obtained only by relaxation, by rejecting the habit of trying to see. The relaxation cannot be obtained by any sort of effort. If by some methods the imperfect eye is made to act like the normal eye, that is, if it can adopt rapid shifting and central fixation, relaxation is automatically produced and the vision is improved. Various methods of relaxation are being described in detail in the succeeding chapters.

Most people, when told that rest or relaxation will cure their eye troubles, ask why sleep does not do so. The eyes are rarely relaxed completely in sleep, and if they are under a strain when the person is awake, that strain will certainly be continued during sleep, to a greater or less degree.

The idea that it rests the eyes not to use them is also erroneous. The eyes were made to see with, and if when they are open they do not see, it is because they are under such a strain and have such a great error of refraction that they cannot see.

The fact is that when the mind is at rest nothing can tire the eyes, and when the mind is under a strain, nothing can rest them. Anything that rests the mind will benefit the eyes. Almost every one has observed that their eyes tire less quickly when reading an interesting book than when perusing something tiresome or difficult to comprehend.

The time required to effect a permanent cure varies greatly with different individuals. In some cases a few minutes, a few hours or a few days are sufficient, and I believe the time is coming when it will be possible to cure every one quickly. It is only a question of accumulating more facts, and presenting these facts in such a way that the patient can grasp them quickly.

Generally persons who have never worn glasses are more easily cured than those who have, and glasses should be discarded at the beginning of the treatment. When this cannot be done, use of glasses may be permitted for a time; but this always delays the cure. Persons of all ages have been benefited by relaxation treatment; but children usually respond much more quickly than adults.

PREVENTIVE METHODS

1. EYELIDS: The upper eyelids should remain downwards, keeping the eye half open without screwing the lids. The diagrams will clearly show the position of the lids. While looking in front or upwards, the upper lid should not be raised but only the chin, that is, the position of the lids should be at all times as at the time of reading.

It can be demonstrated that keeping the lids downwards relieves the strain. Look at the letter 'C' in the chart at fifteen feet distance. Now raise the eyelids as shown in the figure. Note that the blackness of the letter fades. Now raise the chin and bring the lids downwards. Note that the blackness increases.

The wrong position of the lids is generally seen in myopic patients and in those who use glasses and in other cases of defective sight too. Even normal eyes sometimes raise the lids. Generally in cinemas people sit in such a position that they keep the lids raised and that is why many people suffer from discomforts after seeing the cinema.

Lowering the lids gives rest, while raising the lids causes strain. This is a fundamental factor in the cure of most patients. If the patient can keep the lids downwards all the time then soon he is benefited. It is the first thing to understand and practise. Remember that before beginning the practices of relaxation one should make the position of the lids correct and try to maintain it all the time. Do not squeeze the eyes; it is very harmful. Generally myopic patients try to see distant objects by squeezing their eyes.

2. BLINKING: Blinking is the next important fundamental.

The normal eye blinks frequently; it is done so rapidly and gently that we do not notice it. In blinking the main part is played by the upper lid. The upper lid comes a little downwards to cover the pupil and is again raised, while the lower lid moves up with a little contraction of the muscles. The blinking of the normal eye is different from the blinking of the eye with imperfect sight. Blinking of the eye with imperfect sight is usually very irregular and jerky and is accompanied by a strain of the muscles of the eyelids. In cases of imperfect sight an effort is always being made to hold the eye stationary and to stop the blinking.

Blinking can only be done easily and gently when the upper lid remains downwards. Blinking may be done so rapidly that it does not become conspicuous. The normal eye may blink three or four times in one second. When the blinking is done properly, things are seen continuously and they move with a quick jump. Regarding the objects without blinking is an effort, a strain which always lowers the vision.

It is interesting to observe the eyes of some people when they are asleep. One may note that the eyelids are blinking which prevents the eyes from straining or staring, although the persons are quite unconscious of it.

Blinking is a quick method of resting the eyes and can be practised unconsciously all day long, regardless of what one may be doing. Blinking is very simple, and it will be found that a great deal of more reading can be done with blinking than without it, and also the eyes will not be so tired.

Education in Blinking

1. Notice how gently a tiny baby blinks. Now sit in a very comfortable chair. Gently close the eyes and imagine that you are watching a tiny baby blinking. Then gently open the eyes keeping the sight downwards and gently blink. Make frequent blinks without any effort. Remember that the upper lids should not be raised too high and there must not be

any strain, otherwise blinking will turn into winking which is as bad as non-blinking.

2. Count the numbers irregularly (as 4, 1, 3, 6, 9, 13, 15 and so forth) and blink for each count. By consciously blinking correctly, it will in time become an unconscious habit.

3. Place a mirror before you. Look to the right eye and then to the left, blink on each side. It will keep you aware of wrong blinking.

4. Place your folded fingers on your knees and keep the nails of the hands upwards. See the nails of the right hand and blink, then see the nails of the left hand and blink; while doing so move your head from side to side.

5. Take a wrist watch and put it near your ear. Blink at each tick.

6. Walk and blink at each step.

7. Take two pencils one in each hand. Keep one at six inches and the other at one foot from the eyes on the same line. Look at the top of each pencil alternately; you will notice that the lid is raised a little while seeing the distant pencil and lowered while seeing the nearer pencil.
Then close the eyes and imagine as if you are moving your sight from one pencil to another.

Blinking Improves the Vision. Look at the letter 'C' in the chart at a distance of fifteen feet. Now stare and stop blinking; note that the darkness of the letter fades. Now begin to blink and note that the darkness reappears. Take your book. Read without blinking and with blinking and note the difference. You will note that if you do not blink even for a second, the letters become blurred, the vision becomes defective, the eyes are strained; and when you do not blink for hours, you will find that the strain is very much increased. This continued strain causes defective vision.

3. READING: Keep the book at a lower level than the chin so that the lids may not be raised, and hold it at a

distance where the print is quite distinct. Then blink twice at least in reading one line. Do not read in the sun because the glare reflected from the paper causes strain to the eyes. If one at all wants to read in the sun, he should arrange the book in such a way that the sun does not fall on the paper. Reading while lying can also be done without any discomfort if one keeps the head raised and blinks frequently. Reading while lying to the side is harmful. Reading while resting the chin and face on the palm of the hand causes strain. It is a great mistake to stop blinking while reading.

While reading it is useful to shift the sight now and then to a distant object in the room. A few seconds change of focus between the paragraphs or between each page would save many people from common eye strain which causes myopia.

To improve reading with central fixation take a card, preferably of dark colour, having a circular hole cut near the centre, about 15 mm. in diametre. Use the card for a time in ordinary reading, by holding it flat against the reading matter and moving it along. When the card is moved along to the right to allow reading, it will be noticed that the line of words appears to travel to the left.

Fine print reading is supposed to be one of the necessary evils of civilization; but the reading of the fine print, when it can be done without discomfort, has invariably proved to be beneficial and the dimmer the light in which it can be read, and the closer to the eyes it can be held, the greater the benefit. By this means severe pain in the eyes has been relieved in a few minutes or even instantly. The reason is that fine print cannot be read in a dim light and close to the eyes unless the eyes are relaxed whereas large print can be read in a good light and at ordinary reading distance although the eyes may be under a strain. When fine print can be read under adverse conditions, the reading of ordinary print under ordinary conditions is vastly improved. Reading the fine print daily cures presbyopia (old age sight) and many other diseases of the eye which usually occur in old age.

4. READING IN MOVING VEHICLES: Persons who wish to preserve their eyesight are frequently warned not to read in moving vehicles. But since under modern conditions of life many persons have to spend a large part of their time in moving vehicles, and many of them have no other time to read, it is useless to expect that they will ever discontinue the practice. Fortunately the theory of its injuriousness is not borne out by the facts. When the object regarded is moved more or less rapidly, strain and lowered vision are, at first, always produced; but this is always temporary, and ultimately the vision is improved by the practice.

5. WRITING: While writing keep the sight on the point of the pen and move the sight with its movement. A common mistake is to write forward and at the same time to look at the back letters. If one cannot shift the sight according to the pen movement in the beginning, one may draw first straight lines, then angular lines, big letters and small letters. When writing is done rightly, handwriting becomes decidedly better.

Draw a circle about the size of a coin and fill in it with clearly defined dots. The poor sighted will begin with fewer but larger dots. Others begin with twenty, fifty or a hundred or more dots, the objective being to cover the whole area with as many dots as possible. This method helps in developing correct use of the eyes.

6. SEWING: Many women suffer from eye strain while sewing or doing needle-work. They gradually feel headache after working even for a short time. The mistake they commit is that they keep their eyes fixed on their work and blink at long intervals. They should blink frequently and move the sight with the movement of the needle. If the needle comes up, the sight also should move up and when the needle goes down to the cloth, the sight should shift to the cloth. This shifting relieves the strain. In machine work

and in continuous stitching one should blink frequently.

When one finds it difficult to thread a needle follow any of the suggestions:

1. Hold the needle in such a position that white background is visible through the eyelet of the needle.

2. Move the focus around the outline of the eyelet.

3. Move the hands holding the needle and thread slowly and easily about.

4. Keep the head moving slightly.

7. SPINNING: As you move the handle of the spinning wheel in a circular way, move your body also in a circular way gently, without any effort. In the left hand take the cotton piece. As you begin to spin, move your eyes according to the movement of your left hand. When the hand goes to the spindle move your sight to the point of the spindle, and when you remove the hand towards you, shift your sight towards you. It is a general mistake to keep the sight fixed on the spindle. This staring stops blinking, causes headache and dizziness. Spinning gives good relaxation if done methodically.

8. CINEMA: Cinematograph pictures are commonly supposed to be very injurious to the eyes, and it is a fact that they often cause much discomfort and the lowering of vision. They can, however, be made a means of improving the sight. When they hurt the eyes, it is because the subject strains to see them. If this tendency to strain can be overcome, the vision is always improved and if the practice of viewing pictures is continued long enough, many eye troubles are relieved.

Those who have distant sight defective are greatly helped by seeing the same cinematograph pictures more than once. At the first visit one may look at the pictures taking the seat in a place near about the screen in the front rows of seats. On the next visit, take a seat about twenty feet further back. Because of the familiarity, the pictures will be more easily visible than at the first time. The greater familiarity will, on a third visit, permit of further retreat towards the back of the theatre.

How to See a Cinema Picture: Sit erect comfortably, keep your upper lids down while raising the chin and blink frequently.

The common mistake while seeing the cinema is to keep the lids raised and stop blinking.

9. RIDING: While travelling in a train or riding on horseback, move your body according to the movement of the train or horse. Do not be stiff. Imagine that the side objects appear to move backwards. To stop this apparent movement of objects is impossible, and the effort to do so may be very uncomfortable. The greater the effort, the greater the discomfort, and is the cause of headache and nausea. When you ride in an elevator, look at one part of the elevator, imagine that it is moving backwards, avoid looking at the floor.

10. DRIVING: It is interesting to note that people who drive motor cars suffer greatly from eye strain. Taxi drivers are more or less under a nerve strain. Many of them, when they have an accident, believe that it was not their fault. The remedy is to use the eyes in such a way as not to produce a stare. Shift your sight from the speedometer to the centre of the road and notice how the distant road in front comes towards you and finally rolls, as it were, under the car. Keep up blinking and shifting from the near point to the distance. Another way is to imagine the near side objects moving backwards, while the distant side object moving forward. One should keep up blinking frequently. Do not fix the sight on a distant object.

11. HOW TO LOOK AT OBJECTS? The eyes should see as the ears hear without making any effort. While looking at an object, if it is not clear, do not try to make it clear, but shift your sight to other objects. Remember to blink frequently. It is good to shift the sight from one point to the other of the object regarded. Trying to see objects while

moving fastly causes great strain. While in motion, imagine side objects moving backwards. To keep up the imagination of a dot or some other thing, while looking at objects, is very helpful.

12. SNELLEN TEST CARD: Reading a familiar object tends to relax; hence the daily reading of the Snellen test card at about fifteen feet distance is usually sufficient for this purpose. Read the test card first with both eyes and then with each eye separately, covering the other eye with the palm of the hand avoiding any pressure upon the eyeball. Daily reading of the Snellen test card has proved to be an effective method to prevent and cure errors of refraction and other eye troubles. Every home should have a Snellen test card. It is best to place this card permanently on the wall in good light and every member of the family or household should read the card every day.

13. HEARING: Closing the eyes to listen is very helpful. Rest the eyes and deliberately use the ears. Avoid straining to hear but quietly become receptive to sound. The same thing with smell; enjoy the fragrance of a flower while closing the eyes.

Usually people stare directly at the singer or speaker and thus lose the relaxation. How relaxing it is if one keeps his eyes closed while hearing a music or a lecture. A woman having defective eyesight gained normal vision in half an hour time when she tuned herself with her music while keeping the eyes closed and open.

CHAPTER V

SUN TREATMENT AND EYE-BATH

The sun is a wonderful help in relieving all sorts of discomforts of the eyes. The sun is the best help and, in my opinion, no other method can take the place of the sun treatment. The sun is regarded as the god of the eyes by the Hindus, and it is a truth that the sun works like a god for the eyes. The eyes of some people become blind or defective after seeing the solar eclipse; that is because they stare at the sun. Any good method, when practised in a wrong way, may cause harm. I advise every eye patient to enjoy the sun both morning and evening. Our *Rishis* have advised us to offer our prayers daily facing the rising sun. It is also a Hindu rite of worship to throw water on the ground while blinking towards the sun after bath. By facing the sun in a proper manner, the eyes become very bright and shining, attractive and magnetic. The vitality of the eye is greatly increased and no microbe is able to attack the eye. Inflammatory conditions and other discomforts of the eyes are soon cured. In fact, the sun is the *"elixir vitae"* for the eye.

The health of the eye is based on light as the health of the lungs is based on air. The eye is the creation of light. When life first appeared on this planet of ours, it was in the form of protoplasmic cells which had no specific sense organs. It was the action of the environment on the organism which in the course of time made it evolve different organs for its transactions with the outer world. Thus, the light rays of the sun developed the organ of sight, the vibrations of sound developed the organ of hearing and so forth. It is for this reason that we find that not only light rays of the sun are very beneficial to the eyes, but they are also indispensable for their health and activity. Living beings, which usually live underground like earth-worms, have no organs of vision; even animals which possess eyes lose their vision if they are confined for a sufficiently long time in darkness. Fishes living in dark caves become blind; miners generally suffer from defective eyesight and other inflammatory eye troubles. People, who live in the dark and seldom see the sun, like miners, for example, have always something wrong with their eyes. In the houses where the light is poor many children acquire a dislike for the sun light. Some of them keep their eyes covered with their hands, or bury their faces in a pillow and do all they possibly can to avoid the exposure of their eyes to ordinary light. Putting these children in a dark room is a blunder. I obtained best results in the cure of these cases by encouraging the patients to spend a good deal of their time out of doors with their faces exposed to the direct rays of the sun. Not only is the sun beneficial to children, but it is also beneficial to adults.

Of course after remaining in a dark room and suddenly going out into the bright light, one feels the change, and if one is at all nervous, the effect of the light on the eyes is magnified, exaggerated. When such persons are afraid of the light or their eyes are hypersensitive to light, they usually obtain immediate relief from the discomfort by use of dark glasses or an eye-shade. This relief is temporary, and very soon, darker glasses are needed. Eye patients who have used eye-shades habitually, are very difficult to cure. Sun treatment, when used properly in all such cases, is often followed by quick results. Many persons really feel photophobia or glare while going in the sun, although their eyes are quite good. That happens because they keep their eyelids raised and stop blinking. This causes staring which is the cause of the discomfort. Such patients are very easily benefited simply by lowering the eyelids and blinking while going out.

1. SUN TREATMENT WITH CLOSED EYES: Ask the patient

to sit comfortably facing the sun with eyelids closed. The body sways from side to side, gently and lazily. The eyeballs appear to be moving according to the movements of the body. If the eyeballs move in the opposite direction (which can be seen through the closed eyelids), ask the patient to move them with the movement of the head. At first there may be slight discomfort which usually disappears in a few minutes. Now turn the back to the sun or come in the shade, keep the eyes closed and cover them with the palms for five minutes or longer. Then open the eyes and you will notice the relief at once. By repetition the benefit becomes greater and more permanent. This is the safest sun treatment which can be given to every eye patient without causing any kind of discomfort. To sit in the hot sun for a long time causes, sometimes, headache or discomfort in the body. One should at once stop the sun treatment as soon as the sun causes discomfort in the body. It is better to take sun treatment many times for short periods than at one time for a long period. Do not look at the sun with open eyes.

2. WITH CLOSED EYES AND SUN-GLASS: When the eyes become accustomed to face the sun with closed eyelids, use the sun-glass. Focus the light on the closed eyelids, which at first is very disagreeable. The patient continuously moves the body, head and eyes from side to side. The focussed light seems to be moving in the opposite direction. Do not focus the light at one point for more than a second; otherwise you may burn the part. One should be very cautious in giving this treatment.

If this treatment is given properly, one obtains greater benefit than by merely facing the sun with closed eyelids. This treatment is given only for about two minutes at a time. One can give it for more time if the patient does not feel any discomfort.

3. EXPOSURE TREATMENT: Gently lift the upper eyelid towards the brow, exposing some of the white part of the

eye above the pupil. At first, it may be well to shade the
eyes from the sun until the patient acquires sufficient control to look down easily, continuously and without strain.
With the eyes looking far down, one focusses the direct
rays of the sun on the exposed white part of the eye, with
a strong convex glass (sun-glass) moving the glass from
side to side quickly to avoid the heat of the concentrated
sun light. One needs to caution the patient to avoid looking directly at the sun while the light is focussed on the
eye. The length of time devoted to focussing the light on
the white part of the eye should never be longer than a
few seconds.

The results obtained from this method have usually been
very gratifying. When the eyes are inflamed from disease of
the eyelids, the cornea, the iris, the retina, the optic nerve,
from glaucoma and other inflammations, the use of the
burning glass has been followed immediately by a lessening
of the redness and a decided improvement in vision.

Direct sunlight focussed on white part of the eye is
beneficial in many cases of blindness with hardening of the
eyeball (glaucoma), or softening of the eyeball (cyclitis),
also in cases of cataract, and of opacities, of cornea and
in other parts of the eye.

4. WITH OPEN EYES: Looking at the sun with eyes open
is also a very great help to the eyes and is the best way
to enjoy the sun; but one should not take this treatment
without a director. Defective eyes should not enjoy this
treatment unless they have become accustomed to stand
strong sun light with eyes closed. Begin this treatment when
the sun begins to rise, and then stronger sun enjoyed by
and by. Never take this treatment when the sun is hot or
red.

Sway your body, head and eyes from side to side in a
gentle way while looking down. Blink frequently. Then
gently raise the chin bringing the eyes towards the sun. Do
not try to look directly at the sun. While swaying, look at

the sides of the sun and imagine that the sun moves in the
opposite direction. Another way to look towards the sun is
to imagine the nearer objects to be moving in the opposite
direction and the farther objects in the same direction. The
eyes may be closed every now and then.

It is very important to imagine the objects moving in the
opposite direction. If you stop this swing or do not feel,
it means you are staring.

It is good to stand in cold water while facing the sun
with open eyes as the heat rays are quickly absorbed by
water.

5. SUN TREATMENT FOR YOUNG CHILDREN: Hold the
child in such a way that the rays of the sun fall on the
eyes, and move it continuously in slow, short easy curves,
instead of throwing the child rapidly, irregularly and intermittently from side to side. The treatment may be given
for five minutes or more. Very useful in trachoma, conjunctivitis and other eye discomforts of the child's eyes.

6. SUN TREATMENT WHILE WALKING: Keep the sight on
the ground and walk facing the sun. Imagine the road and
side objects moving backwards.

7. ALTERNATE SUN GAZING: Looking at the morning sun
for a few seconds and then palming for half a minute gives
the exercise to the iris by alternate contraction and dila-
tation of the pupil. The retina is stimulated by light and
relaxed by darkness. This alternate light and dark adapta-
bility for 5 to 10 minutes is very helpful in many cases of
defective eyesight and chronic iritis.

GENERAL DIRECTIONS ABOUT SUN TREATMENT

1. Do not sit in the sun when it is hot. Morning and
evening are the best times for sun treatment. During summer it is very helpful to dip the feet in cold water and
cover the head with a cloth while taking sun treatment. In

winter, one can take the sun treatment (first method) at any time.

2. Begin sun treatment with the mild rays of the sun, that is, the mornings and the evenings, and gradually the strong rays of the sun may be taken.

3. Sun treatment, according to the first method described before, can be taken by anybody without any hesitation, but other kinds of sun treatment should not be taken without the presence of an experienced director.

4. While moving the head from side to side, remember that the eyes should move in the direction of the head. Remember to blink while gazing at the sun.

5. When the sun is not shining, substitute a strong electric light. A 1,000-watt electric light is preferable, but requires special wiring; however, a 200 to 300-watt light can be used with benefit, and does not require special wiring. Sit about six inches from the light, or as near as you can without discomfort from the heat, allowing it to shine on your closed eyelids as in the sun treatment.

6. After sun treatment it is good to wash the eyes with cold water.

7. The vision should remain clear after taking sun treatment. If there is dimness after sun treatment, it indicates strain. Relieve it by palming and swinging.

8. If you face the sun for five minutes daily, it is sufficient to keep your eyes healthy.

9. All eye patients can take the sun treatment whether they use any medicine or not.

10. Demonstrate that the sun treatment gives immediate benefit in many diseases of the eye.

Before the treatment, take a record of your best vision on the Snellen test card or Reading test types with both eyes together and each eye separately without the glasses. Then sit in the sun with your eyes closed, slowly moving your head a short distance from side to side, and allowing the sun to shine directly on your closed eyelids. Forget about your eyes; just think of something pleasant and let your mind drift from one pleasant thought to another. Then come to your former place. Before opening your eyes, palm for a few minutes. Then test your vision and note the improvement.

EYE-BATH

Eye-bath is very effective in toning up the eyes and the surrounding tissues. It causes relaxation and helps in improving the eyesight. Taken after sun treatment, it adds to the relief and relaxation. Cold water should be used for eye-bath. A weak solution of common salt or *triphala* water, or Ophthalmo can also be used.

DIRECTIONS FOR TAKING EYE-BATH

1. Fill the cup nearly to its brim and put it against the eye gently. Keep the eyes downwards and go on blinking with both the eyes. Wash each eye for two minutes. Do not keep the eye-cup against the eye for too long a time, as that may produce suction which is not desirable. It should be removed and reapplied several times after every 20 or 30 seconds.

2. Dip your hands in the bowl (palms upwards and cupped), and raise them full of water to within two inches of your eyes. Then splash the cold water on your eyes smartly, but not violently. Repeat this about twenty times, then dry the face and the eyes. It is a very good thing to do whenever the eyes feel tired.

3. Fill a basin with cold water. Dip your face. Keep the eyes open and blink. Take out the face to breathe. Repeat ten times or more. After removing the face from water each time, you may look at the sun with open eyes for a few seconds and again dip the face in water. The sun rays

do not harm the eyes; because there is a layer of cold water in front of the eye and the heat rays are soon absorbed by cold water.

CHAPTER VI

RELAXATION METHODS

CENTRAL FIXATION

When the normal eye sees a thing, it sees only that part of the thing best on which it fixes itself and the other parts not so well. This is called Central Fixation.

The retina of the eye has a point of maximum sensitiveness called fovea centralis, and the eye sees best through this point. The result is that the part of an object regarded is seen best. This quality of the eye is called Central Fixation. When the sight is normal or the mind is at perfect rest, the sensitiveness of the fovea is normal, and the eye sees best where it looks at; but when the sight is imperfect, from whatever cause, the sensitiveness of the fovea and central fixation are lowered, so that the eye sees other parts or objects not directly regarded equally well, or even better, with other parts of the retina. For example, here are two letters C.O. While C is regarded, it is seen better and clearer than O and when O is regarded, it is seen clearer and better than C. This is central fixation. But if while regarding C, O is seen equally well or even better then it is lowered central fixation or eccentric fixation.

When the eye possesses central fixation it not only possesses perfect sight, but it is perfectly at rest and can be used indefinitely without fatigue. Loss of central fixation means strain, and when it is habitual leads to all sorts of abnormal conditions and is, in fact, at the bottom of most eye troubles. By improving central fixation the vision soon begins to improve, but the limits of improvement depend upon the degree of central fixation. Not only do all errors of refraction and all functional disturbances of the eye disappear when it sees by central fixation, but many organic conditions are relieved or cured. I am unable to set any limits to its possibilities. The benefits of central fixation already observed are, in short, so great that the subject merits further investigation.

The smaller the thing or letter regarded in this way, or the shorter the distance the patient has to look away from a letter to another letter in order to see the first indistinctly the better is the Central Fixation. Central Fixation is perfect when the eye is able to regard a very small point better than another such point placed by its side.

While regarding a letter or an object the eye shifts from one point to another rapidly and continuously; it does not fix itself on one point for more than a fraction of a second. If it tries to do so, it begins to strain and loses its central fixation. This can readily be demonstrated by trying to hold one part of a letter before the eye for an appreciable length of time. No matter how good the sight, it will begin to blur, or even disappear, very quickly, and sometimes the effort to hold it will produce pain. In the case of a few exceptional people a point may appear to be held for a considerable length of time; the subjects themselves may think that they are holding it, but this is only because the eye shifts unconsciously, and the movements from one part to another are very rapid.

Why does the eye see best where it fixes itself?

The retina or the image-receiving plate has a point of maximum sensitiveness, and every other part is less sensitive in proportion as it is removed from that point. This point of maximum sensitiveness or of best vision is called the "Fovea Centralis" literally meaning the "Central pit". The eye with normal vision, therefore, sees best one part of everything at which it looks, and everything else worse. When the sight is normal the sensitiveness of the central pit is normal, but when the sight is imperfect, from whatever cause, the sensitiveness of the pit is lowered, so that the eye sees equally well, or even better with other parts of the retina.

If the eye does not see best where it fixes itself how to account for it?

The eye with normal sight never tries to see. It does its function without any effort as other sense organs do. An effort to see is the underlying cause of loss of central fixation. Whenever the eye tries to see, it at once ceases to have normal vision. A person may look at the stars with normal vision, but if he tries to count the stars in any particular direction he will lose central fixation and probably become myopic, because the attempt to do these things usually results in an effort to see. A patient was able to look at the letter K on the Snellen test card with normal vision, but when asked to count its twenty-seven corners he lost central fixation and the letter could not be seen.

According to the degree of an effort to see, the sensitiveness of the fovea or Central Fixation is affected; the patient can no longer see best the point which he is looking at but sees the objects not directly regarded as well or better, because the sensitiveness of the retina has now become approximately equal in every part, or is even better in the outer parts than in the centre.

It requires a strain to fail to see at the distance, because the eye at rest is adjusted for distant vision. While the eye is at rest if one does anything in order to see at the distance, one inevitably does the wrong thing. The shape of the eyeball cannot be altered during distant vision without strain. It is equally a strain to fail to see at the near point.

PERFECT CENTRAL FIXATION or perfect sight is impossible unless the eye shifts continually from point to point and such shifting is a striking illustration of mental control necessary for normal vision. It requires perfect mental control to think of thousands of things in a fraction of a second; and each point of fixation has to be thought of separately, because it is impossible to think of two things or two parts of one thing, perfectly at the same time. The eye with imperfect sight tries to accomplish the impossible by looking fixedly at one point for appreciable length of time, that is, by staring. When it looks at a strange letter and does not see, it keeps on looking at it in an effort to see it better. Such efforts always fail, and are an important factor in the production of loss of central fixation and imperfect sight.

When the eye possesses central fixation it shifts rapidly from one point to the other of a letter or an object and it always sees the previous point of fixation worse.

When the eye regards a letter either at the distance or at the near point, the letter may appear to pulsate or move in various directions. When it looks from one letter to another on the Snellen test card, or from one side of a letter to another, not only the letter, but the whole line of letters and the whole card, may appear to move from side to side. This apparent movement called swinging is due to the shifting of the eye, and is always in a direction contrary to its movement. If one looks at the top of a letter, the letter appears to move downward. If one looks at the bottom, the letter appears to move upward.

The eye having central fixation possesses perfect sight and can be used indefinitely without fatigue. It is open and quiet; no nervous movements are observable. The letters on the Snellen test card are seen perfectly black and perfectly distinct and they do not have to be sought. The white centres inside the letters called haloes seem to be whiter than the margin of the paper. The eye maintains perfect gentle blinking.

On the contrary, when the eye does not possess central fixation, it ceases to shift rapidly and to see the point shifted from worse, the sight ceases to be normal, the swing being either prevented or lengthened or reversed. The eye quickly tires, and its appearance, with that of the face, is expressive of effort or strain. The letters on the test card are not seen very black and very distinct, they are sought and chased. The eye goes after them. An effort is made to see them.

What is Eccentric Fixation?

Eccentric Fixation is the opposite of "Central Fixation". The eye does not see best where it is looking. For example, there are two letters on the chart R and B, if the eye sees R on the chart, R is not seen better than B while B is seen equally well or better than R. This condition is sometimes so extreme that the patient may look as far away from R as it is possible to see it, and yet see R just as well as when looking directly at it.

Eccentric Fixation is a symptom of strain and even in lesser degrees it is so unnatural that great discomfort, or even pain, can be produced in a few seconds by trying to see every part of an area three or four inches in extent at twenty feet or even less, or an area of an inch or less at the near point, equally well at one time. This strain, when it is habitual, leads to all sorts of abnormal conditions and is, in fact, at the bottom of most eye troubles. The discomfort and pain may be absent, however, in the chronic conditions, and it is an encouraging symptom when the patient begins to experience them.

In most cases of eccentric fixation the eye quickly tires and the eyeball makes irregular movements. In some cases these irregular movements are so extensive and sufficiently marked that they resemble nystagmus (a condition in which there is a conspicuous and more or less rhythmic movement of the eyeball from side to side). The eye stares and stops gentle blinking or it blinks at long intervals with jerks and effort.

While reading if the eye experiences pain or discomfort, it indicates that the eye tries to see many words at a time and suffer from eccentric fixation. Persons, who avoid reading fine print and prefer big prints, usually suffer from eccentric fixation because in large print the eye tries to look at a larger area at one time. Similarly in writing if one feels pain or discomfort, it is because one loses central fixation and the eye tries to see the word or letter that is being written and the back words or letters already written at one time. When the eye keeps up central fixation, it shifts itself with the movement of the pen and does not try to see the back words or letters already written.

How does central fixation help in improving defective sight and mental faculties?

In all cases of defective sight, sensitiveness of the central spot is more or less decreased, the rays are distorted, and the eye is not able to see best where it is looking. When the sensitiveness of the central spot is improved by central fixation exercises given in this book, the rays are centred, the vision and the health of the eye are improved.

Since central fixation is impossible without mental control, the central fixation of the eye means central fixation of the mind. It means, therefore, health in all parts of the body, for the mind has a great influence on the operations of the physical mechanism. Not only the sight, but all the other senses—touch, taste, hearing and smell—are benefited by central fixation. All the vital processes—digestion, assimilation, elimination, etc. — are improved by it. The symptoms of functional and organic diseases are relieved. The efficiency of the mind is enormously increased.

In what diseases is central fixation most helpful?

In very high myopia, where glasses do not improve the vision and reading has become difficult; in Hypermetropia, Presbyopia or old age sight, Astigmatism, Early Glaucoma, Early Cataract, Nystagmus and Retinal diseases; in choroiditis and all cases who feel difficulty and discomfort in reading; and in acquired Nightblindness and Colour blindness.

SUGGESTIONS FOR
CENTRAL FIXATION EXERCISES

1. For all patients, it is good to have the following pro-gramme of practices morning and evening:—

(a) First have sun treatment. Sit facing the sun with the eyes closed and head covered for 5 minutes. While sitting in the sun move the body gently from side to side like a pendulum.

(b) Then come to the shade, wash the eyes and face with cold water, and sit down comfortably for 5 minutes to practise palming. By palming I mean to close the eyes gently and cover them with the palms of the hands in such a way as to avoid any pressure on the eyeballs. When all the light is shut off by palming, one should experience all perfect dark before the eyes as if one is in a perfect dark room. If it is not perfect dark before the eyes in palming and some other colours appear, it indicates that eyes and mind are under a strain. To relieve this strain imagine something perfectly black or some pleasant object as a flower, a boat floating in the river, clouds moving in the sky, etc. Some persons like to remember familiar things, thus a knife is remembered by a surgeon, dollies by girls, babies by mothers. When the imagination is perfect accord-ing to the reality, one sees all perfectly dark before the eyes when the eyes are closed and covered.

(c) Then open the eyes gently; blink and practise central fixation practices.

In blinking the lids, make a gentle movement. The upper lid comes a little down and then is again raised.

The upper lid should not touch the lower lid. Look at the normal eyes and learn blinking.

(Application of Resolvent 200 in the eyes with a rod just before sun treatment gives better results).

2. Keep the upper lids downwards and blink gently and frequently.

3. Note that the part of the object regarded is seen darker and clearer.

4. While shifting the sight from one object to another, move the head also along with the sight.

5. Keep the book at a distance from where you see it best and subsequently the distance may be increased in myopic patients and decreased in hypermetropic and presbyopic patients.

6. Frequent palming helps central fixation.

7. Feeling of strain or discomfort indicates wrong practice. Stop and practise palming or swinging.

8. Practice first with both eyes and then with each eye separately, covering the other with the palm of one hand avoiding any pressure on the eyeball.

9. Before beginning central fixation exercise, test the sight of both eyes and each eye separately, on the Reading Test Type Fundamentals at 9 or 12 inches and keep the record.

10. Central fixation may be practised mentally also while keeping the eyes closed.

Practice No. 1

Keep the sight on the white centre of the letter "O" in Fig.1. Blink gently. Note that the white centre seems to be whiter than the rest of the whole page. Further, note that the blackness of the letter "O" is darker than the other "O" (Fig.2) which is within the field of vision. Close the eyes for a second and imagine "O". Repeat till you note the facts. Then shift your sight to "O" (Fig.2) and note that now white centre flashes whiter and its outline darker than the other "O" (Fig.1). Close the eyes for a second and repeat ten times.

The ability to imagine the white centre whiter can be acquired by the memory of white snow, white paint or anything perfectly white, with the eyes closed for a part of a minute. Then, when the eyes are opened, the white centre is imagined or seen much whiter than before.

Fig. 1　　　　　　　　　　Fig. 2

PRACTICE NO. 2

Look at the first dot or "O" and note that it is darker and clearer than the dot or "O" which is placed by its side. Close the eyes for a second, again open and note that the dot or "O" is clearer and darker than before.

Now look at the next dot or "O" placed by the side of the first one, and practise in a similar way.

Then practise on the smaller pairs. Should the bigger dots and O's distract the mind, they may be covered.

PRACTICE NO. 2

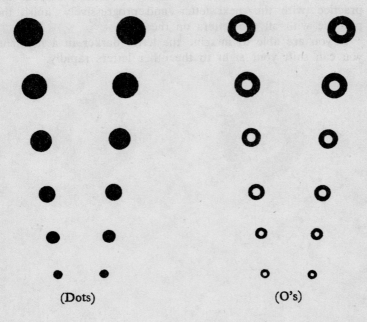

(Dots)   (O's)

PRACTICE No. 3 (DIAL CHART)

Look at one letter in the dial chart given on the next page and note that it is blacker and clearer than all the other letters. Close the eyes for a moment, then open the eyes and shift your sight to the next letter on the dial. Note as before that it is blacker and clearer than the others. Repeat the practice with the next letter and progressively finish the practice with all the letters on the dial.

If you are able to imagine the letter darker in a moment, you can shift your sight to the other letters rapidly.

Practice No. 3

Y Q C P 3 D F S N O E R T G D V

DIAL CHART

PRACTICE NO. 4

Practice of central fixation on Om chart is very useful because one does central fixation on the thick and thin outline of the character.

(*a*) Keep your sight at the point where ॐ begins and note that this portion of the ॐ is seen darker than the rest of the ॐ. Move your sight gradually on the rest of the ॐ, noting all the time that the portion of the ॐ seen becomes darker, thus making the whole character ॐ of a darker shade.

Close the eyes, imagine ॐ as you did with the eyes open. Repeat ten times with both eyes opened and closed.

(*b*) There is a circle all around the ॐ, and around the circle are angular lines; move your sight from one end to the other of one of these lines and note that the line seen is the darkest. Close the eyes and imagine as instructed. Repeat the same with the other lines.

(*c*) Over the ॐ is an arc and there is a small dot above the arc ˘. With each blink shift your sight from one end of the arc to the other end.

Note that the black dot seems to be moving in the opposite direction. Close the eyes; move your sight on the arc in your imagination and note the movements of the dot. Alternate with open and closed eyes.

PRACTICE NO. 4

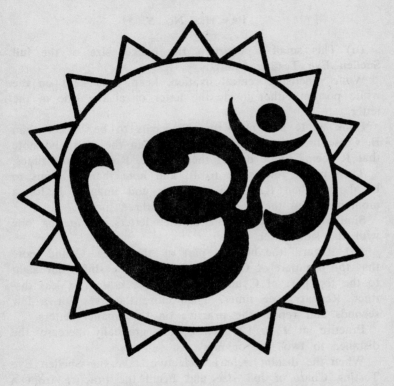

**This OM chart for Eye Exercises
was found on Bhojpatra in Kashmir.**

PRACTICE NO. 5

(a) This small C chart is the pocket size of the full Snellen Eye Testing Chart.

While practising central fixation, keep your sight on the white portion either inside the letter or at the side of the letter.

Look at R and note that R seems to be darker than B. Close the eyes and imagine R. Open the eyes and note that R seems to be darker than before. Repeat three times.

Then move your sight to B, and note that B seems to be darker than R. Close the eyes and imagine B for a moment. Open the eyes and repeat three times.

Similarly, practise on the smaller letters, comparing one with the side letter.

(b) Regard the bottom part of the letter C and note that the top part of C is less distinct, then shift your sight to the top part of C and note that the bottom is less distinct. Repeat three times. Then close the eyes for a few seconds and repeat the practice on the smaller letters.

Practise at 9 or 12 inches, then gradually increase the distance to two feet or more.

When the distant sight is defective, take the Snellen Eye Testing Chart of full size and begin the practice from a distance of 2 feet, and gradually increase the distance of the chart to 10 feet or more.

Similar practices are done on the Pot-Hook card.

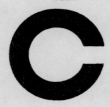

50 FEET

C

30 FEET

RB

20 FEET

TFP

15 FEET

5CGO

10 FEET

4KBER

5 FEET

3VYFPT

4 FEET

2QCOGD☐C

3 FEET

RZ3B8SHKFO

Snellen Test Card — Pocket Size

PRACTICE No. 6

Pot-Hook Card is usually meant for children. Let the child sit at five feet or more from this E card. Request him to make a picture of the characters, or he may indicate by finger which way each 'E' points.

Shift the sight on each arm of E and note that the arm of E regarded appears more distinct than the other arms.

100

50

20

15

10

5

4

3

Pot-Hook Card

PRACTICE No. 7

READING OF FUNDAMENTALS

First move your sight on the white lines in between the lines of fine print from No. 7 to 14. Now read from No. 1, blink gently and frequently and move the head a little along with the sight. Close the eyes for a minute after reading each fundamental.

Read it at a convenient distance, then gradually decrease the distance to 6 inches if you are presbyopic or hypermetropic and increase the distance to 9 or 12 inches if you are myopic.

At night read it under a candle light.

Fundamentals

By
W. H. Bates, M. D.

1. Central Fixation is seeing best where you are looking.

2. Favourable conditions: Light may be bright or dim. The distance of the print from the eyes, where seen best, also varies with people.

3. Shifting: With normal sight the eyes are moving all the time.

4. Swinging: When the eyes move slowly or rapidly from side to side, stationary objects appear to move in the opposite direction.

5. Long Swing : Stand with the feet about one foot apart, turn the body to the right—at the same time lifting the heel of the left foot. Do not move the head or eyes or pay any attention to the apparent movement of stationary objects. Now place the left heel on the floor, turn the body to the left, raising the heel of the right foot. Alternate.

6. Drifting Swing : When practising this swing, one pays no attention to the clearness of stationary objects, which appear to be moving. The eyes wander from point to point slowly, easily, or lazily, so that the stare or strain may be avoided.

7. Variable Swing : Hold the forefinger of one hand six inches from the right eye and about the same distance to the right, look straight ahead and move the head a short distance from side to side. The finger appears to move.

8. Stationary Objects Moving: By moving the head and eyes a short distance from side to side, being sure to blink, one can imagine stationary objects to be moving.

9. Memory: Improving the memory of letters and other objects improves the vision for everything.

10. Imagination: We see only what we think we see, or what we imagine. We can only imagine what we remember.

11. Rest: All cases of Imperfect sight are improved by closing the eyes and resting them.

12. Palming: The closed eyes may be covered with the palm of one or both hands.

13. Blinking: The normal eye blinks or closes and opens very frequently.

14. Mental Pictures: As long as one is awake one has all kinds of memories of mental pictures. If these pictures are remembered easily, perfectly, the vision is benefited.

PRACTICE NO. 8 (Reading of Fine print.)

Fine print reading or reading of Photographic type reduction is a benefit to the eye. If you read it daily, your near or reading sight will ever remain perfect and you will be saved from cataract, glaucoma or other old age diseases of the eyes.

If you feel any difficulty in reading it, first take sun treatment for five minutes, then wash the eyes with cold water and palm for 5 minutes.

When one imagines the white spaces perfectly white, the print becomes very black and legible, apparently of its own volition.

Exercise 1 — Shift the sight on the white line of fine print and blink at each line.

2 — Read fine print in good light and candle light alternately.

3 — Read fine print and glance at the blank surface alternately.

4 — Read fine print and the Snellen eye chart placed at ten or twenty feet alternately.

PRACTICE No. 8

Seven Truths of Normal Sight

1. Normal Sight can always be demonstrated in the normal eye, but only under favorable conditions.
2. Central Fixation: The letter or part of the letter regarded is always seen best.
3. Shifting: The point regarded changes rapidly and continuously.
4. Swinging: When the shifting is slow, the letters appear to move from side to side, or in other directions with a pendulum-like motion.
5. Memory is perfect. The color and background of the letters or other objects seen, are remembered perfectly, instantaneously and continuously.
6. Imagination is good One may even see the white part of letters whiter than it really is, while the black is not altered by distance, illumination, size, or form, of the letters.
7. Rest or relaxation of the eye and mind is perfect and can always be demonstrated.

When one of these seven fundamentals is perfect, all are perfect.

Specimen of Fine Print

CHAPTER XIII

MEMORY AS AN AID TO VISION

WHEN the mind is able to remember perfectly any phenomenon of the senses, it is always perfectly relaxed. The sight is normal, if the eyes are open; and when they are closed and covered so as to exclude all the light, one sees a perfectly black field —that is nothing at all. If you can remember the ticking of a watch, or an odor or a taste perfectly, your mind is perfectly at rest, and you will see a perfect black when your eyes are closed and covered. If your memory of a sensation of touch could be equal to the reality, you would see nothing but black when the light was excluded from your eyes. If you were to remember a bar of music perfectly when your eyes were closed and covered, you would see nothing but black. But in the case of any of these phenomena it is not easy to test the correctness of the memory, and the same is true of colors other than black. All other colors, including white, are altered by the amount of light to which they are exposed, and are seldom seen as perfectly as it is possible for the normal eye to see them. But when the sight is normal, black is just as black in a dim light as in a bright one. It is also just as black at the distance as at the near-point, while a small area is just as black as a large one, and, in fact, appears blacker. Black is, moreover, more readily

Photographic Type Reduction

Patients who cannot read photographic type reduction are benefited simply by looking at it.

PRACTICE NO. 9

1. Read this Reading Test Type chart from below upwards. Glance at the white centre of the letter regarded and observe that the letter appears darker and clearer in this way.

2. Read it in good light and candle light alternately.

3. Copy this chart in the notebook.

4. Walk and read this chart while blinking at each letter, slowly and lazily.

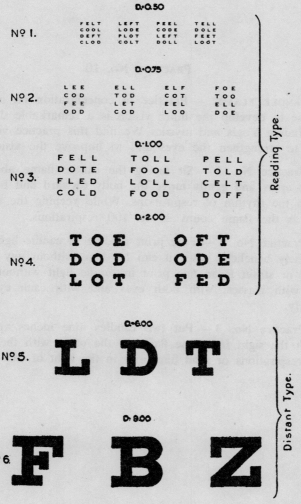

Reading Test Type

PRACTICE No. 10

CANDLE FLAME: — Practice of concentration on a candle flame to develop the inner vision is a remarkable discovery of Indian Yogis and mystics. We find this practice very useful to strengthen the eyes and to improve the vision.

Practice No. 1 — Sit facing the candle flame about one foot apart and gently move the body forward and backward with the rhythm of respirations. While keeping the sight towards the flame count 25 to 100 respirations.

Practice No. 2 — Fine print reading in candle light is extremely beneficial when it can be done without any discomfort or strain. Read fine print in candle light without glasses or with glasses, with both eyes and with each eye separately.

Practice No. 3 — Put two candles nine inches apart and shift the sight from one flame to the other with the rhythm of respirations or read fine print in the light of two candles.

PRACTICE NO. II
READ THE NATURAL WAY

I. First, adjust the distance of the printed matter to the eyes. When one sees the print best one has arrived at the correct distance.

2. It has been observed that readers keep the book at arms length which is about eighteen inches, but on care-full observation they find that keeping the book closer makes the print clearer. Usually to the normal eye the reading distance is within the range of ten to twelve inches.

3. The second factor is that the head and eyes should move together while reading. In many instances it will be found that the head is fixed, and only the eyes move along the printed line. Because of this the eyeball slants, and the letter observed is not in the direct line of vision. This causes fatigue and strain and headache, double-vision, even squint.

4. The eye in its natural state is a moving organ. When it is made to stare fixedly, rigidity and tension of the eyeball and eyelids result. Blinking easily will not be possible and thus the eye will be unable to throw off fatigue. Reading in bright light is to be avoided because the glare reflected from the paper causes strain. Light just sufficient to read is enough. Reading in candle light has been found soothing.

5. It is a fallacy that large print aids eyesight and memory. The eye has to see a larger area at a time while reading large print and hence there is greater strain. It has been observed that fine print aids eye-sight because there is less strain involved and so there is no fatigue. Printed matter is a field of black and white. It is found that reading is comfortable and less taxing to the eyes when the sight is directed along the white space between the letters, or white space immediately below them. By contrast, the black print images are sharper and clearer. Shifting the body from side to side or backward and forward makes it easier to train to this habit.

CHAPTER VII

PALMING

Every one must have noticed that when the eyes are tired, closing the eyes for a moment clears the vision and a kind of relief is felt in the eyes. But as some light still comes through the closed eyelids (move your hand before the closed eyes and you will notice the movements of the hand), a still greater relief can be obtained by excluding this light as well. This is done by covering the closed eyes with the palms of the hands (the fingers being crossed upon the forehead) in such a way as to avoid pressure on the eyeball. This practice is called "palming". When the eyes with normal sight are closed and covered so as to shut all the light, the retina does not receive any light and the result is that one sees or experiences perfect black. Palming is one of the best methods for relieving strain and securing relaxation.

Q. What is the effect of palming?

The effects of a successful palming are:—

1. One sees or experiences a perfectly black field before the eyes.

2. There is a definite improvement in the eyesight when the eyes are opened after palming and the improvement is lasting; there is a cooling or soothing sensation in the eyes; strain, pain or headache, which may have been there before palming, disappear completely; one feels rest and relaxation in the eyes as well as in the mind and in the body.

The effects of imperfect palming are:—

1. One does not see or experience a perfect black field before the closed eyes but may be able to see an approximate black. Patients who fail to see even an approximate black when they palm, state that instead of black they see streaks or floating clouds of grey, flashes of

light, patches of red, blue, green, yellow, white, etc. Sometimes clouds of black will be seen moving across the field. In other cases the black will be seen for a few seconds then some other colour will take its place. The different ways in which patients can fail to see black when their eyes are closed and covered are, in fact, very numerous and often very peculiar.

2. When the eyes are opened the improvement in sight is either partial or nothing at all and the improvement does not last long. One does not feel a perfect relaxation. The greater the degree of the relaxation produced by palming the more of it is retained when the eyes are opened and the longer it lasts.

3. Mental strain is the sign of imperfect palming.

Why should one experience a perfect black field before the eyes in Palming?

If you go to a room where there is no light you will see that the room is quite dark. Similarly when there is no light entering the eyes in palming, one sees a perfect black field before the eyes. The retina of the eye reacts only to light, and when there is no light it does not do its function of receiving the images of objects. When the retina stops its function one sees all perfect dark.

If one does not see perfect black in palming, what is its cause and its remedy?

Mental or bodily strain is the cause of imperfect palming. Even if the eyes are closed so as to exclude all the light the visual centres of the brain may still be disturbed and instead of seeing black, the patients will see various illusions of lights and colours. When the mind is able to remember perfectly any phenomenon of the senses, it is always perfectly relaxed; and one sees a perfectly black field — that is nothing at all If one can remember the ticking of a watch, or an odour or a taste perfectly, one's mind is perfectly at rest, and he will see a perfect black when the eyes are closed and covered. If one can remember the colours of objects perfectly he would see nothing but black. Memory of black objects is usually more helpful than the objects of other colours.

For successful palming glance at a letter of the Snellen Test Card or black velvet for a second and immediately close the eyes for about half a minute. Repeat till the memory of black is equal to sight.

Or first practise central fixation on the letters of the Snellen Eye Chart and then do palming.

What class of patients are not able to do palming perfectly?

Generally the worse the condition of the eyesight, the greater the imperfection in imagination while palming. Yet some persons with imperfect sight are able to palm almost perfectly from the beginning, and are, therefore, very quickly cured. Any disturbance of mind or body, such as fatigue, hunger, anger, worry or depression, also makes it difficult for patients to see black when they palm. Persons who can see perfect black under ordinary conditions are often unable to do so without assistance when they are ill or in pain.

Some patients were so impressed with the vividness of the colours which they imagined they saw that no amount of argument could convince them that they did not actually see them with their eyes. If other people saw bright lights or colours, with their eyes closed and covered, they admitted that these things were illusion; but what they themselves saw under the same conditions was a reality. They would not believe until they had themselves demonstrated the truth, that their illusions were due to an imagination beyond their control.

What are the signs of perfect palming?

1. When palming is perfect the colour of any object remembered is remembered perfectly and one feels perfectly relaxed and one sees a perfect black field before the eyes when they are closed and covered.

2. When the eyes are opened perfect sight comes in-

stantaneously and the letters on the chart are perfectly black and are distinctly recognized. If good vision is obtained only after a second or two, the palming is said to be imperfect.

3. The white centres of the letters called haloes seem to be whiter than the margin of the chart.

SUGGESTIONS

1. Sit comfortably. Close the eyes gently and cover them with the cups of palms in such a way that there is no pressure on the eyeballs.
2. Tuck a pillow or cushion below the elbows or rest them on a table so that the elbows may not be tired. A piece of black velvet may be placed on the pillow.
3. Generally people like to palm for 5 to 10 minutes. The longer some people palm the greater the relaxation they obtain and the darker the shade of black they are able both to remember and see. Others are able to palm sucessfully only for short periods, but begin to strain if they keep it up too long. During summer if the eyes feel heat or if the palms perspire one may put thin wet cold cotton pads on the palms and then practise palming.
4. Palming can be practised at any time. It is necessary for patients with bad eyesight to practise palming several times a day. It is helpful to palm after sun treatment.
5. It is impossible to succeed by effort to concentrate on the black.
6. While palming, imagination of black is more helpful than that of other colours. Some particular kind of black objects may be found to be more easily remembered than others. Black plush of a high grade for instance, could be more easily remembered by many persons as compared with black velvet, silk, ink, letters on the test cards.

7. Familiar black objects can often be remembered more easily by the patient than those that are less so. A dressmaker, for instance, was able to remember a thread of black silk when he could not remember any other black object.

8. Patients often say that they remember black perfectly when they do not. One can usually tell whether they can actually remember a perfect black by noting the effect of palming on the vision. If there is no improvement in the sight when the eyes are opened, it can be demonstrated, by bringing the black colour to the patient, that it has not been remembered perfectly.

9. Although a large majority of patients are helped by palming yet there are some who are unable to see black, and only increase their strain by palming. The method should be dropped in such cases, and other relaxation methods should be practised to improve the sight.

10. When black objects are not convenient to remember, imagine some other objects which have been seen perfectly or clearly, or something pleasant such as a flower, a boat floating in the river, clouds moving in the sky etc., and let the mind drift from one thought to another. Familiar objects as a hammer by a carpenter, a brush by an artist, a knife by a surgeon, etc., are remembered easily. Little girls like to remember their dollies. Mothers like to remember their babies.

11. Before beginning to practise palming for the improvement of eyesight it is better to test the vision both for the distance and the near point and keep the record for comparison.

12. Washing the hands immediately before palming proves beneficial. After palming when you open the eyes remember to blink gently and frequently.

13. One should discard the glasses if one is really anxious to improve the vision. It is a wrong belief that one will

get strain if he discards the glasses. If the patient keeps up blinking and practises palming frequently, no strain can occur and the sight will steadily improve. Those who are unable to discard the glasses from the very beginning for any reason, may reduce the power of the glasses gradually, and use them only when necessary; but this always delays the cure.

14. Time: Palming may be practised at any time. To improve the vision, morning time is the best; but practise palming four or five times in the course of the day whether with the chart or without it. It will give you relaxation for the whole of the day. Bad cases require the practice of palming five to ten times a day. Palming before going to bed induces sound sleep. Whenever you feel your eyes tired or you are excited or feel headache or want to remember something, just palm for a few minutes. One should not practise palming with the chart to improve his sight when there is any disturbance of the mind or the body, such as fatigue, noise, hunger, anger, worry, or depression. These conditions make successful palming difficult.

Children should practise before going to school, or at the beginning of the school work. This will keep their mind at rest and they will be able to follow the lessons easily.

PRACTICE

1. Sit comfortably. Place the Snellen Eye Testing Chart in good light at a distance from where you can read the first four lines of the chart quite clearly. Now palm for five minutes or more. After palming remove the hands and open the eyes gently but keep up gentle blinking. Look at the white centres of the letters of the fourth line one by one noting that the white centre flashes whiter than the margin of the chart. The

black area of the letter will automatically be seen blacker than before. Now move your chair backwards by six inches, repeat alternately palming and glancing at the white centres. Increase the distance gradually to 20 feet. When the fourth line is easily seen at 20 feet distance, come nearer to a distance from where the fifth line can be read. Repeat palming and go on increasing the distance to 20 feet. Similarly repeat on the sixth and seventh lines also.

While blinking and glancing at the white centre of the letter one may note that the letter makes short movements in any direction. Do not try to stop these movements.

If the patient is a child and does not understand glancing at the white centre of the letter, let him read the letters one by one with blinking or he may close the eyes after reading each letter. The rest of the process is to be repeated as described.

2. After practising palming take the chart in the hand. Look at the top part of the first letter C on the Snellen Test Card. Note that the bottom part which you are not regarding, but which is seen also while you are looking at the top of the letter, seems to be less distinct than the top. Now look at the bottom part and note that the top is seen less distinct. Close the eyes for a few seconds. Repeat the process three times. Then practise on other letters till you are able to practise on the seventh line 2, Q, C, O, of the test card.

Now place the chart at a distance from where you can read fourth line 5, C, G, O. Practise palming again and repeat the above exercise either from the first letter of the chart or from the first letter of the fourth line. Go on increasing the distance to twenty feet. Then come nearer from where you can read the fifth line, and so on.

3. While palming imagine the drill of F, given below and then practise on the chart as above.

 Drill of F.—"There is a letter F on the test card. Imagine that F stands at attention like a soldier and is perfect black. Now he starts his drill. His two arms are pointed to the right when he begins. Imagine the arms moving to the left and back. Then one arm is pointed to the left and one to the right and F becomes a T! Both arms are then stretched up forming a Y."

4. While palming hear some story, music, gramophone or radio, and then practise on the chart. One patient was benefited by hearing the story of a black ant while palming. This black ant came out of the dark soil and climbed up to the stem of a beautiful rose. It was slow work with the ant, but it kept on climbing, going on to the extremity of the first branch and then to another crawling to the extreme tip of every leaf until it finally located the flower. It crawled with great labour over the petals until it found deep down in the centre of the rose a little white cup filled with honey. The patient could picture the ant carrying off some of the honey, crawling to the top of the flower and then down back to the stem, finally meeting another ant on the ground, with whom she had a short talk with much gesticulating of head and feet. Then the second ant started off on the same journey. The patient, while palming, listened very attentively to this talk, which was drawn out for seven minutes.

5. If the reading sight is defective, practise on the reading test type after palming. Hold the reading test type at a distance from where it can be seen best. First move the sight on the white spaces in between the lines of print, and then begin to read with gentle blinking. If the eyes feel a strain or if the letters begin to fade, at once close the eyes and repeat palming. Sometimes it is helpful to move the pencil or the

tip of the finger below the words while reading.

Gradually increase the distance of the test type up to twelve inches if you are myopic, and decrease the distance of the test type up to six inches if you are hypermetropic or presbyopic. A person with normal vision usually holds the chart or book at a distance of 9 to 12 inches.

6. Cover a table with a black or green cloth, preferably velvet, rest the elbows on the table and palm. Then release one of the hands from palming, keeping the eyes closed and shaded with the other hand. With the fingers of the free hand roll a ball on the table and imagine the eyes following it. This kind of exercise has an advantage of directing the thoughts upon form and is useful for those who cannot imagine in an abstract way. Then gently open the eyes and glance at white centres of letters of the chart while blinking or read the Reading test type.

7. After palming practice on a view card or scenery. Select a view card or a picture in colour or black and white. Start to see the picture at first its near objects and then look at its far objects and set the mind and sight somewhere between near and far objects. Make no effort but glance in a natural way. Observe that the flatness of the picture initially seen becomes three-dimensional. The details of the picture become sharply visible. Suddenly the whole picture appears very beautiful and absorbs the mind in its seeing. For example, take a view card of Taj Mahal Agra, it will begin to appear as if a real monument wonderfully beautiful. The mind and eyes will be felt greatly relaxed. After seeing the picture if you read the eye chart, the vision will be found improved.

CHAPTER VIII

MEMORY AS AN AID TO EYESIGHT

The mind keeps the remembrance of many things which were formerly seen. This remembrance of things is called memory. We remember things consciously or unconsciously, with the eyes closed as well as with the eyes open. When the memory of a letter or other object is according to the reality, it is called a perfect memory; and when the memory of a letter or other object is not according to the real object, it is called an imperfect memory.

When the memory of the colour of the object is perfect, the mind is perfectly relaxed, and perfect sight is the result when the eyes are open; and when the eyes are closed and covered so as to exclude all the light, one sees all perfectly dark before the eyes. The memory of black colour gives a correct idea of relaxation. If the colour of blackness is remembered perfectly, one is perfectly relaxed. If it is remembered imperfectly or cannot be remembered at all one has very little or no relaxation.

Why is the memory of a black object to be preferred to the memory of other colours?

All other colours, including white are altered by the amount of light to which they are exposed and are seldom seen as perfectly as it is possible for the normal eye to see them. But when the sight is normal, black is just as black in a dim light as in a bright one. It is also just as black at the distance as at the near point, while a small area is just as black as a large one. Black is, moreover, more readily available than any other colour. There is nothing blacker than printer's ink. By means of the memory of black, therefore, it is possible to measure accurately one's own relaxation.

Although black is, as a rule, the best colour to remember some patients are bored or depressed by it, and prefer to remember objects of white or some other colour. A familiar object, or one with pleasant associations, is often easier to remember than one which has no particular interest. One patient was cured by the memory of a yellow butter cup, and another was able to remember the opal of her ring when she could not remember any black object. Whatever the patient finds easiest to remember is the best to remember, because memory can never be perfect unless it is easy.

What is the effect of memory on the eye?

When the memory is perfect, the sight is normal. The eyes and mind are free from strain, and their function is passive and quite natural. A letter on the chart is seen perfectly black, and perfect darkness is realized when the eyes are closed and covered. But when the memory is imperfect, the eyes and mind are under a strain and they make an effort to see; the sight is also imperfect.

If one with imperfect sight can improve the memory of black or some other colour or can realize all perfectly dark when the eyes are closed and covered, the strain is relieved and the relaxation is experienced. The sight is improved. In the treatment of functional eye troubles the relationship between relaxation and memory is of great practical importance. The eyes and mind may not show any symptoms of strain. Those who strain most often suffer the least discomfort. But by means of his ability to remember black the patient can always know whether he is straining or not, and is able, therefore, to avoid the conditions that produce strain.

What is the test of a perfect memory?

Patients may measure the accuracy of their memory by remembering a small black dot or full stop.

1. When the memory of the dot or of any other thing is perfect, it is instantaneous. If a few seconds or longer are necessary to remember it, the memory is never perfect.

2. A perfect memory is not only instantaneous, but continuous.

3. When the memory is perfect, perfect sight comes instantaneously. If good vision is obtained only after a second or two, it can always be demonstrated that the memory is imperfect also.

4. The memory of the dot is a test of relaxation. It is the evidence by which the patient knows that his eyes and mind are at rest. It may be compared to the steam gauge of an engine, which has nothing to do with the machinery, but it is of great importance in giving information of the ability of the mechanism to do its work. When the dot is black, one knows that the engine of the eye is in a good working order. When the dot fades, or is lost, one knows that it is out of order, and requires treatment.

How should one improve the memory of a black dot or a letter or an object?

The memory of a black dot or a letter or an object is to be improved both with the eyes closed and open, but no effort is needed to remember. As the relaxation improves the memory also improves, because it is obtained only during moments of relaxation, and retained only as long as the causes of strain are avoided.

For most patients palming provided the most favourable conditions for the memory of black. When the strain to see is lessened by the exclusion of light, the patient usually becomes able to remember black for a few seconds or longer, and this period of relaxation can be prolonged by one of the two ways:

(a). Open the eyes and look at a dot or a letter on the Snellen Test Card with central fixation at the distance at which it can be seen best, and then palm.

(b). While palming shift mentally from one black object to another, or from one part of a black object to another. After palming open the eyes and look at a blank surface as a wall, without trying consciously to see and keep up the memory of the dot in the mind. If successful, the vision is improved. But if, with the improved vision, details upon the surface begin to come out or if the patient begins to think of the test card which he has seen imperfectly, the strain to see will return and the memory of the black dot will be lost.

How will you help the patients who feel difficulty in remembering black objects?

They are directed to look at the black objects — letter on the chart, black cap, black paint, etc. — at a distance at which the colour can be seen best. Then close the eyes and remember the colour. Again open the eyes and look at the black object. Repeat this until the memory becomes spontaneous and appears to be equal to the sight. While still holding the memory of black they should cover the closed eyes with palms of the hands. If the memory of the black is perfect, the whole background will be black. If it is not, or if it does not become so in the course of a few seconds, the eyes should be opened and the black object regarded again.

How can one improve the imagination of black if it comes for a few seconds and then soon fades away?

Patients who are unable to remember black for more than a few seconds are helped by central fixation. Look at the black object, shift the sight from one part to another or from one object to another, noting that the part regarded is seen best; then remember with the eyes closed the part regarded best. It is impossible to see, remember, or imagine, even for a second, without shifting the sight from one part to another, or to some other object and back again; and the attempt to do so always produces strain. Those who think they are remembering a black object continuously are unconsciously comparing it with something not so black, or else its colour and position are constantly changing. When a patient does not shift the sight unconsciously, he must be encouraged to do so consciously. He may be directed, for instance, to remember successively a black hat, a black shoe, a black velvet dress holding each one not more than a fraction of a second. Many persons have been benefited by remembering in turn all the letters of the alphabet perfectly black.

In some cases the following method has proved successful:

One should remember a black curtain or a black background and a piece of starch or white paper on this background and imagine that on the starch there is the letter F as black as the background. Now let the starch or paper go away and remember only the F on the black background. While remembering F, shift mentally from one part of F to another. This process can be repeated many a time.

If with the eyes open it is not possible to see black perfectly, how can one remember black perfectly with the eyes closed?

Any condition of the eye which prevents the patient from seeing black perfectly makes palming difficult. In such cases it is usually best for the patient to improve his sight by other methods before trying to palm. Blind persons usually have more trouble in seeing black than those who can see, but may be helped by the memory of a black object which was familiar to them before they lost their sight. A painter who saw grey instead of black letters, became able to see black by the aid of memory of black paint.

The following method is helpful in such a case:— Let the patient regard a letter on the Snellen Test Card at the distance at which the colour is seen best, then close his eyes and remember it. If the palming produces relaxation, it will be possible to imagine a deeper shade of black than was seen, and when the eyes will be opened the letter can be seen blacker than it was at first. A still deeper black can then be imagined and seen by repetition. The patient may be helped to remember at times some objects other than black.

What are the conditions when one fails to have perfect memory of a black dot?

1. When one makes an effort to remember a black dot.
2. When one tries to imagine the dot on other objects instead of simply remembering it in the mind.
3. When the mind and eyes are under a strain on account of staring, partly closing the eyes or screwing, frowning etc.
4. When one tries to see all the letters of a line equally well at one time or when one makes an effort to see the letters or other things.
5. Excitement of various kinds, unexpected noise and unusual occurrences, worries, anxieties and physical discomforts also affect the memory.
6. Speaking of or thinking about unpleasant things or telling a lie.

SUGGESTIONS

1. The smaller the area of black which the patient is able to remember, the greater is the degree of relaxation indicated. Some patients find it easier, at first, to remember a somewhat larger area, such as one of the letters on the Snellen Test Card with one part blacker than the rest. They may begin with the big C, then proceed to the smaller letters, and finally get to a small black dot or full stop. It is then found that this small area is remembered more easily than the larger ones, and that its blackness is more intense. Some patients find it easier to remember a punctuation mark, a colon for instance, with one part blacker than the other parts. As it is impossible for the mind to think of one thing continuously, some patients find it useful in the beginning to shift consciously from one of these black areas to another, and to realize the swing or pulsation produced by such shifting. When the memory becomes per-

fect, one object may be held continuously in the mind without conscious shifting, while the swing is realised only when attention is directed to the matter.

2. When there is no time to practise on the Snellen Eye Chart, the memory of a black dot or an object is sufficient, and one can remember the dot at any hour of the day or night, whatever the patient may be doing.

3. Memory of a black dot relieves pain. The sense of taste, smell and hearing are also improved, while the efficiency of mind is increased. A patient had severe pain in her head for many days. She was directed to look at a large black letter, note its blackness, then cover her closed eyes with the palm of her hands, shutting out all the light, and to remember the blackness of the letter until she saw everything black. In less than three minutes she said, "I now see everything perfectly black. I feel no pain in my head. I am completely relieved, and I thank you very much."

4. You may not be aware of a strain, and apparently there may be no symptom of a strain present; but still you might be under strain, by means of the ability to remember black you can always know whether you are straining or not, and in this way you can avoid the conditions that produce a strain.

5. When the memory is very imperfect, central fixation exercises and palming prove very helpful to improve the memory.

6. If the eyes or head pain while remembering a dot or an object, give up the practice, because it is being done with effort. Relieve the pain by swinging exercises or palming.

EXERCISES

Exercise 1
(a) Look at a dot or a fullstop at a distance where it is

seen best, then close the eyes and remember it. Repeat several times till the memory of the dot is equal to the dot seen with open eyes. When successful the dot seems to be making short movements in various directions in the imagination. Any attempt to stop the movement of the dot will fail the memory.

(b) Then open the eyes and look at the ground or a blank wall keeping up the memory of the dot. If the memory of the dot begins to fade, close the eyes and remember it again. By repetition the dot will be remembered with eyes open also.

(c) When the memory of the black dot with open eyes is perfect, place the Snellen test card on a white wall at ten feet distance or nearer. Now remember a black dot while looking a little to one side of the test card, say, a foot or more; then look a little nearer to the test card and finally look between the lines of letters. In this way one may become able to see the letters without losing the memory of the black dot. When one can do this one may become able to go a step farther, and look directly at a letter without losing control of the memory of the dot.

Exercise 2

Remember the black dot and look at the bottom part of the letter on the Snellen test card. See or imagine the black dot as part of the letter, while noting that the rest of the letter is less black and less distinct than the part directly regarded. When one can do this one becomes able to remember the dot better than when the letter is seen all alike.

While imagining the dot as a part of the letter, the patient notes whether the bottom of the letter is straight, curved, or open, without losing the dot on the bottom of the letter. When he can do this, he is asked to do the same with the sides and top of the letter, still holding the dot on the bottom.

Exercise 3

Look at your signature and then close the eyes while remembering it. It is easy to remember one letter of the signature better than the whole word. When the memory of the letter with the eyes closed is perfect, keep up its memory with the eyes open.

When successful, look at the white space below the letter of the chart which is placed at ten feet or nearer. When this is done, look at the bottom part of the letter still holding the memory of the letter.

Instead of a letter or dot, one may remember the face of a friend, a certain picture, the odour of a rose, or the tune of some song.

Exercise 4.

Some patients get negative images with the eyes closed, that is, when they remember a black letter a white letter appears in the imagination. Such cases may adopt the following method.

Look at a letter of the Snellen Test Card at a distance from where it is seen best, for part of a minute; then close the eyes for a second. By repetition with the eyes open and closed, the mental picture becomes more frequent and lasts longer. The practice may be begun from bigger to smaller letters.

When the memory of a black letter improves practice on the Snellen Test Card while keeping the letter in the memory.

Exercise 5.

Take a pointer five feet long. A coloured pointer with black and white paints at intervals of twelve inches is preferable. Stand about five feet away from the chart. Look at the top letter of the chart and point it, close the eyes while holding the rod in position. Make a clear image of the letter in your mind then flash a glance to where you know the pointer is touching that letter. Close the eyes quickly and repeat; both eyes together then each eye separately. When the letter is clear and distinct, lower your pointer to a smaller letter and practise again. You will find that the letter or part of the letter you are pointing to, and actually looking at, appears blacker and clearer than the rest.

CHAPTER IX

IMAGINATION AS AN AID TO VISION

IMAGINATION: We see very largely with the mind, and only partly with the eyes. The phenomena of vision depends upon the mind's interpretation of the impressions upon the retina. What we see is not that impression, but our own interpretation of it. This interpretation of the mind or thinking of the mind is called imagination. The following are some of the examples.

1. Take a Snellen test card and hold it at a distance from your eyes at which your sight is fairly good. Look at the white centre of the large 'O' and compare the whiteness of the centre of the 'O' with the whiteness of the rest of the card. You may do it readily; but if not, use a screen, that is, card with a small hole in it. With that card, cover over the black part of the letter 'O' and note the white centre of the letter which is exposed by the opening of the screen. Remove the screen and observe that there is a change in the appearance of the white, which appears to be whiter, when the black part of the letter is exposed. When the black part of the letter is covered with a screen, the centre of the 'O' is of the same whiteness as the rest of the card. It is, therefore, possible to demonstrate that you do not see the white centre of the 'O' whiter than the rest of the card, because you are seeing something that is not there. When you see something that is not there, you do not really see it, you only imagine it.

2. The moon looks smaller at the zenith than it does at the horizon.

3. When you see a large letter of the Snellen test card, the part regarded appears blacker than it really is.

4. A portrait painted by one painter may look entirely different from a portrait of the same person by some other

artist.

5. A drawing may be made of a plaster cast which may appear all right when first completed, but may show many faults when studied by the same artist at other times.

6. In a totally dark room, one often imagines that he sees a white ghost. The imagination may be so vivid that no amount of argument will convince him that he did not see a ghost.

Thus our sight depends upon our imagination or the mind's interpretation of the retinal image. The white centres of the letters on the Snellen test card are imagined by the normal eye to be whiter than the other parts of the card while the eye with imperfect sight imagines the white centres of the letters to be less white than the margin of the card, or imagines them to be of the same shade. So when the sight is imperfect, not only the eye is at fault but the imagination is also impaired. In short, when the eye is out of focus, the mind is also out of focus.

What is the difference between memory and imagination?

Imagination is closely allied to memory, although distinct from it. When you think of an object of which you have the memory, it is imagination. Imagination depends upon the memory, because a thing can be imagined only as well as it can be remembered. You can not imagine a sunset unless you have seen one; if you strain to imagine a blue sun, which you have never seen, you will become myopic. You cannot imagine a cat unless you have its memory.

What is the relation between memory, imagination and sight?

Neither imagination nor memory can be perfect unless the mind is relaxed. Therefore when the imagination and memory are perfect, the sight is perfect. Imagination, memory and sight are, in fact, coexistent. When one is perfect, all are perfect; and when one is imperfect, all are imperfect. For example, look at the letter 'O' and note that the white centre appears whiter, and the black outline appears blacker than the rest of the letters. What you have seen, you can remember and imagine also. The whiter one can remember and imagine the centre of 'O' the better becomes the vision of the letter 'O', and when the vision of the letter 'O' improves, the vision of all the letters on the test card improves. The perfect imagination of the white centre of the 'O' means perfect imagination of the black, because one cannot imagine the white perfectly without imagining the black perfectly.

Persons with normal vision use their memory, or imagination, as an aid to sight. When persons with imperfect sight improve the imagination of the white centres of the letters, the sight is also improved by the aid of improved imagination.

We can remember perfectly what we have seen perfectly.

We can imagine perfectly what we can remember perfectly.

We can see perfectly what we can imagine perfectly.

What is the effect of imagination on eyesight?

If you imagine a letter perfectly, you will see that the letter and other letters in its neighbourhood will come out more distinctly; because it is impossible for you to relax and imagine perfectly and at the same time strain and see a letter imperfect.

Imagination, when used properly, is the most satisfactory, most accurate, most helpful method that we know of to obtain perfect sight. If our imagination for something or for the small letter 'O' or a black dot is as good at twenty feet, forty feet, sixty feet, or further, as it is at a near point where we see it perfectly, our vision is just as good as our imagination. The perfect imagination of the letter 'O' or of other objects is always associated with perfect sight of other letters or objects not known.

How should one improve the imagination if it is defective?

Methods which improve the memory will improve the imagination also. The following method improves the imagination in most of the cases:

Look at the white spaces in between the lines of print. The white spaces will appear whiter than the margin of the page. If they do not appear whiter, remember something very white as whitewash or a white pillow etc. Seeing the white spaces improves the imagination, and the vision for the letters is also improved. One can improve the vision for reading not by looking at the letters, but by improving the imagination of the white spaces. To look at the letters very soon brings on strain, with imperfect sight. To look at the white spaces and to improve their whiteness, is a benefit to the imagination and to the vision. By practice one becomes able to imagine or to see the white spaces more perfectly—the better the imagination, the better the sight. Similarly look at the white centres of the letters on the Snellen test card instead of seeing the black area of the letters.

SUGGESTIONS

1. Encourage patients by saying "Do not try to see the letter. Imagine that what you see is perfectly black with a very white space. What we see is simply our imagination."

2. Making an effort to see or imagine lowers the vision.

3. Convince the patient that the only way of perfect sight is by rest or relaxation. When sight is imperfect, a strain is there to keep it imperfect.

4. Imperfect imagination produces all sorts of errors of refraction, and may even produce organic changes in the eyeball. One can, by imagining a letter imperfectly, increase the hardness of the eyeball. Imagination of a letter seen perfectly softens the eyeball in glaucoma with great benefit to the pain and the imperfect sight. All errors of refraction are cured temporarily or permanently by the imagination of a perfect sight.

COMPARISONS

In practising with the Snellen Test Card, when the vision is imperfect, the blackness of the letters is modified and the white spaces inside the letters are also modified. By comparing the blackness of the large letters with the blackness of the smaller ones, it can be demonstrated that the larger letters are imperfectly seen.

When one notes the whiteness in the centre of a large letter, seen indistinctly, it is usually possible to compare the whiteness seen with the remembered whiteness of something else. By alternately comparing the whiteness in the centre of a letter with the memory of a better white, as the snow on the top of a mountain, the whiteness of the letter usually improves. In the same way, comparing the shade of black of some other object may be also a benefit to the black.

Most persons with myopia are able to read fine print at a near point quite perfectly. They see the blackness and whiteness of the letters much better than they are able to see the blackness of the larger letters on the Snellen Test Card at 15 or 20 feet. Alternately reading the fine print and regarding the Snellen Test Card, comparing the black and white of the small letters with the black and white of the large letters, is often very beneficial. Some cases of myopia have been cured very promptly by this method.

All persons with imperfect sight for reading are benefited by comparing the whiteness of the spaces between the lines with the memory of objects which are whiter. Many persons can remember white snow with the eyes closed whiter than the spaces between the lines. By alternately closing the eyes for a minute or longer, remembering white snow, white starch, white paint, a white cloud in the sky with the sun shining on it, and flashing the white spaces without trying to read, many persons have materially improved their sight and been cured.

THIN WHITE LINE

The imagination of a thin white line between the lines of print helps in relieving most of the eye troubles. Most people suffering from presbyopia and hypermetropia (long sight) are cured when they become able to imagine that they see this white line brighter and clearer than the margin of the page. It gives a restful, pleasant feeling to all the nerves of the body when the thin, white line is seen, remembered or imagined. In cases of inflammation, when one is able to imagine the thin white line, pain in the eyes, head or other parts of the body disappears as though by magic. Patients with early cataract who become able to imagine this thin white line perfectly very soon become able to read the fine print without effort or strain, and the cataract always improves or becomes less. Patients with astigmatism, squint, diseases of the retina and optic nerve are benefited by the memory or the imagination of the thin white line.

A great many people are very suspicious of the imagination of the thin white line and feel or believe that things imagined are never true. The more ignorant the patient, the less respect he has for his imagination. It comes to them as a great shock to discover that the perfect imagination of the thin white line improves the sight.

The ability to imagine the white line is acquired by the memory of white snow, white paint or anything perfectly white, with the eyes closed for a part of a minute. Some patients count thirty while remembering some white object or some scene with the eyes closed. Then, when the eyes are opened for a second, the white lines are imagined or seen much whiter than before. By remembering perfectly white with the eyes closed and opening them for a few seconds, the vision or the imagination of the white line improves. One needs to be careful not to make an effort to regard the black letters. When the white line is remembered with the eyes closed and with the eyes open, the black letters are read without effort

or strain. Many people discover that they can imagine a
thin line where the bottom of the letters comes in contact
with the white line. The thinner the white line imagined, the
whiter it becomes and more perfectly the letters are read.
Of course, the eyes have to shift from the thin white line
to the letters in order to see them, but the shifting is done
so rapidly, so continuously, so perfectly that the reader does
not notice that he is continuously shifting. When the vision
of the thin white line is imperfect, the shifting is slow and
imperfect, and the vision for the letters is impaired.

HOW TO IMAGINE THE WHITE LINE

1. Hold the card in your hand at ten inches. Move your
sight from one corner to the other of the white lines, without trying to read. While moving the sight keep a short
swing of the body.

2. Blink at each end.

3. Imagine that the line moves in a direction opposite to
that of the swing of the body.

4. Now close the eyes, keep the swing, imagine the white
line or some other object.

5. Then open the eyes and look at the white lines.
Repeat.

EXERCISES

1. LETTER IN THE AIR: Take two similar Snellen test cards.
Place one at a distance of ten feet or less where it cannot
be readily distinguished and appears blurred, and the other
card at a distance of one foot or less, from where you can
see it best. Now regard a letter of the distant card, then
look at the same letter on the card that is near. Then close
the eyes and with your finger draw the same letter in the
air as well as you can remember it. Open your eyes and
continue to draw the imaginary letter with your finger while

looking for only a few seconds at the blurred letter on the card at ten feet or less. Then close your eyes again and remember the letter well enough to draw the letter perfectly in your imagination with your finger. Alternate drawing the letter at ten feet in your imagination with your eyes closed as well as you see it at one foot or nearer. When you can draw the letter as perfectly as you remember it, you see the letter on the distant card in flashes.

By repetition, you will become able not only to imagine always the known letter correctly, but to see it actually for a few seconds at a time. You cannot see a letter perfectly unless you see one part best, that is, by central fixation. Note that you obtain central fixation while practising this method, *i.e.,* you see one part best. Drawing the letter with your finger in your imagination enables you to follow the finger in forming the letter, and with the help of your memory, you can imagine each side of the letters best, in turn, as it is formed. When the letters on the distant card become distinct and clear, then increase the distance of the distant card by two to six inches only. By and by increase the distance to fifteen or twenty feet.

By this method, the memory and the imagination are improved, and when the imagination becomes perfect, the sight is perfect. This method should be practised at least for one hour, twice or thrice, daily. You can benefit highest degrees of myopia, hypermetropia, astigmatism, optic atrophy, progressive cataract, glaucoma, detachment of the retina and other diseases by this method.

2. LETTER IMAGINATION: If the patient is unable to see letters on a certain line of the test card, he is told what the first letter is and is directed to close his eyes and imagine that letter for about ten seconds, then to open the eyes and regard the letter. When the letter is imagined perfectly enough, other letters on that line are seen. Then imagine the first letter of the next line, and so on. If no letter is seen on a certain line, the patient may come to the test

card, see, go back and imagine. By alternately regarding the letter with the eyes open and closed, the imagination of the letter improves in flashes.

By continuing to alternate, the flashes improve and last longer and the vision becomes gradually improved.

3. F. EXERCISE: If you do not get any improvement by practising at fifteen feet distance, bring the card closer to six feet or nearer. Hold another card in your hand and look at the letter 'F' of the ten feet line. See it with a slow, short easy swinging with "F" for a few minutes. Then glance at the first letter of each line of the Snellen's card at the distance of six feet without modifying or stopping the swing of your body. When the vision is improved at six feet, increase the distance by and by till you reach fifteen feet, practising in the same way.

4. Place the Snellen eye chart at a distance where you see it best. Look at the white centre of the letter 'C'. Note that the white centre flashes whiter than the margin of the card, and the whiteness seems to be raised, and the white portion appears in form of a flash. Similarly, the whiteness of other letters is imagined. Gradually increase the distance of the chart. Each time practise upto the seventh line 2, Q, C, O line.

5. IMAGINATION TEST: Place the back of the Snellen test card towards the patient ten feet away from him, and the face of the second card towards him at twelve feet. Both cards can be so arranged that the patient can observe an open space between the two about four or five inches in width.

When the patient moves the head and eyes to the left, the space between the two cards becomes less and one can imagine the nearer card moving to the right, while the more distant card with its letters appears to move to the left.

When the head and the eyes move to the right, the nearer card appears to move to the left, the space becomes larger between the two cards and the patient can imagine the face of the more distant card moving to the right.

Then close the eyes, swing and imagine the nearer card to be moving in the opposite direction, and the more distant card to be moving in the same direction. Repeat. In some cases of defective sight, the nearer card moves in the opposite direction while the distant card may also move in that opposite direction, or it may stop or move in an irregular, jerky manner.

When the imagination of black dot or some object is correct with the eyes closed, the swing of the more distant card becomes normal, the card moves from side to side in the same direction as the head and eyes, and moves slowly, easily, and continuously. The converse is also true, that when the distant card does not move with the head and eyes, the imagination of the object is imperfect.

By the continued practice of this method, the flashes of improved vision become frequent and last longer. Some patients are benefited by practising this method with the eyes closed for a longer time than with the eyes open.

6. Place the eye chart at about 5ft. distance and look at the letters easily with frequent blinking for about 3 seconds. Then close the eyes and mentally shift your imagination on the letters for a few seconds. Repeat several times. A few minutes practice during the day proves very helpful in improving the sight. The value of this practice is increased by focussing strong light on the chart, and the light is switched on with the opening of the eyes and similarly switched off as the eyes close.

CHAPTER X

SHIFTING AND SWINGING

SHIFTING: Moving the eyes from one point to another is called shifting. If you move your hand from one place to another, you are said to be shifting your hand. In the same way, if you look at 'C' on the chart and then see another letter, it means you are shifting your eyes from one point to another. Shifting may be done from side to side, from above downwards, or in any other direction. Horizontal shifting is done more often than other forms of shifting.

SWINGING: When the eyes shift slowly or rapidly from one point to another of the object, the stationary object appears to move in the direction opposite to the movement of the head and eyes. For example, shift your sight from R to B and B to R on the Snellen test card; note that the letters appear to move in a direction contrary to the movement of the eyes. This apparent movement of the object is called swinging. A simple example of the swing is that experienced in a moving train. When you travel in a train, which is moving fast, and look out of the windows, you see the telegraph poles and other objects moving in an opposite direction.

Is it necessary to shift the sight?

When the normal eye has normal sight, it is always shifting from one point to another. The normal eye is never stationary. This is true of the eyes closed as well as of the eyes open. It is impossible for the eye to fix a point longer than a fraction of a second. If it tries to do so, it begins to strain and the vision is lowered. Look at a letter for an appreciable length of time, and note that the letter begins to blur, or even disappear.

The eye gets rest only when it is moving; and when it is moving, it imagines consciously or unconsciously the stationary objects to be moving in the opposite direction. Place your fingers lightly on the closed eyelids, you will feel the eyes to be moving slowly or rapidly in all directions. The swing is as essential to men as to animals. The tiger, the lion and other animals move most of the time while they are awake, and are in this way relaxed. The elephant sways his bulky body from side to side, because it rests him. It is always interesting to watch soldiers march, and observe the sway of their bodies in unison with the rhythm of music. A mother, who is busy with her household work, is always, grateful for the few minutes of rest and relaxation which she gets when rocking the baby. If the heart stops beating, which is really a sway inside the body, the blood has no longer a chance to flow nor the pulse to beat. If the pendulum of the clock stops, the clock does not tell time.

What is the difference between shifting of the eye with normal vision and that of the eye with imperfect vision?

The shifting of the eye with normal vision is rapid and usually not conspicuous. The shifting of the eye with imperfect sight, on the contrary, is slower, and the movements are jerky and made with effort indicating a staring expression.

Therefore, one of the best methods of improving the sight is to imitate consciously the unconscious shifting of normal vision and realize the swinging produced by such shifting. When the sight is imperfect, shifting, if done properly, rests the eye as much as palming, and always improves the sight.

What are the long and short shifting and swinging? What are their benefits.

When the eye shifts more than an inch, it is called a long shift; and when it shifts less than an inch, it is called a short shift. Similarly according to the shift, the swing will be long or short.

The long shift or swing relieves eye discomforts and pain, and helps one to obtain the short swing. The short shift or swing improves the vision. The shorter the shifting and swinging, the better the results in the improvement of the vision. The short swing is more difficult, but when it is successfully practised, one obtains greater amount of relaxation than can be obtained from the long swing. A very long shift or swing — as much as three feet or more — is helpful to those who cannot accomplish a shorter one. When the patient is capable of a short shift or swing, the long shift or swing lowers the vision. In a very short shift, it is not always easy to be conscious that the eye really moves.

What is the cause of failure to realise a swing while shifting?

The cause of failure to produce a swing is strain. Some people try to make the letters swing by effort. Such efforts always fail. The eyes and mind do not swing the letters or other objects; they swing of themselves. The eye can shift voluntarily; but the swing comes of its own accord when the shifting is normal. Swinging does not produce relaxation, but is evidence of it.

It is possible to shift without improvement; but it is impossible to produce the illusion of a swing without improvement. When swinging can be done with a long shift, the movement can gradually be shortened until the patient can shift from the top to the bottom of the smallest letter on the Snellen Test Card or elsewhere and maintain the swing. Later he may become able to be conscious of the swinging of the letters without conscious shifting.

Different people will find various methods of shifting more or less satisfactory. If any method does not succeed, it should be abandoned after one or two trials and something else tried. It is a mistake to continue the practice of any method which does not yield prompt results. The cause of the failure is strain, and it does no good to continue the strain.

SUGGESTIONS

1. When the eye shifts from one point to another, it always sees the previous point of fixation worse as explained in the chapter of central fixation; and it realizes swinging of the object.

2. While shifting the sight from one point to another, if the eyes do not see the previous point of fixation worse, the swing is either prevented or lengthened or reversed. These facts are the keynote of the treatment of shifting and swinging.

3. Shifting and swinging can be practised both with eyes open and closed. For most patients swinging with eyes closed is easier at first than visual swinging. By alternating mental with visual swinging and shifting, rapid progress is sometimes made.

4. Shifting and swinging, as they give the patient something definite to do, are often more successful than other methods of obtaining relaxation, and in some cases remarkable results have been obtained simply by demonstrating to the patient that staring lowers the vision and shifting improves it.

5. After resting the eyes by closing or palming, shifting and swinging practices are often more successful.

6. Shifting and swinging exercises are usually performed on the Snellen eye chart for the improvement of eyesight. When it is not possible to practise with the Snellen Test Card, other objects may be utilized. For instance, one can shift from one window to the other or from one part of a window to another part of the same window, or from one side of an object to another; but in each case produce the illusion that the objects are moving in a direction contrary to the movement of the eye. When reading a book or newspaper, one can shift consciously from one word or letter to another, or from one part of a letter to another.

7. Shifting may be practised slowly or rapidly according

to the state of the vision of the patient. At the beginning, he is likely to strain if he shifts too rapidly; and there will be no swing. The speed can be increased gradually. It is usually impossible, however, to realize the swing if the shifting is more rapid than two or three times a second.

Children like to be swung round or to run around a chair or to ride a rocking horse. Dancing is an excellent exercise that can be taught to children as unconsciously stationary objects appear to move in the opposite direction.

8. WRONG WAYS OF SHIFTING.

1. To turn the head and the body in a direction opposite to that of the eyes, that is, to turn the head to the right while the eyes are turned to the left, or to turn the head to the left while the eyes are turned to the right. Or to turn the body to the right while the head and the eyes are turned to the left, or to turn the body to the left while the head and the eyes are turned to the right.

2. To keep the sight fixed on an object while the head is moving.

3. To move the eyes more irregularly, that is, a longer or shorter distance than the movement of the head.

4. To imagine that the stationary objects do not move in the direction opposite to that of the eyes and the head.

5. To imagine that all the objects or letters seen are of equal clearness.

6. To stop blinking.

9. RIGHT WAY OF SHIFTING: The right way to shift is to move the eyes from one point to another slowly, regularly, continuously, restfully, easily, without effort, without trying to see. The normal eye with normal sight has the habit of always moving or shifting, usually an unconscious habit. When, by practice, the eye with imperfect sight acquires the conscious habit of shifting, the habit will become unconscious afterwards. It often happens that, when one consciously

or intentionally shifts in the wrong way, a better knowledge of the right way to shift may be acquired. When the eyes are moved to the right, stationary objects should appear to move to the left; and when the vision is good, all objects not regarded are seen less distinctly than those regarded. Blinking is very necessary with each shift.

10. YOU WILL FAIL TO REALISE A SWING—
   1. When you feel absolutely certain that the stationary object is always stationary and no movement can be expected.
   2. When you stare at the objects.
   3. When you stop blinking or blink very rapidly.
   4. When the background is not prominent. Suppose you stand before a window and practise swinging. If the background seen through the window is not prominent, you may not be able to imagine the bars of the window to be moving in the opposite direction.
   5. A common mistake that is made is to turn the head to one side and turn the eyes in the opposite direction while swinging.

11. HINTS FOR SUCCESSFUL SWING—
   1. Do not stare at objects and make no effort to see them. Lazily shift your sight from one point to another without having any idea that you are seeing the objects.
   2. The background should be prominent.
   3. If one eye is bad, practise first with the good eye.
   4. Blink once on each side.
   5. Imagine the movement of a pendulum and sway like that.
   6. Move your head, eyes and body rhythmically from side to side.
   7. While practising swing with eyes open, close them for a minute or two after every five minutes.

SHIFTING & SWINGING PRACTICES

These are seven practices. It is better to begin from the first exercise. Keep the lids and the chin in the right position and blink frequently, while practising. The eighth exercise brings prompt results when practised properly.

PRACTICE NO 1. Stand with the feet about one foot apart, facing a window having vertical bars or before a swing stand. Take a long step to the right and note that the bars have gone to the left. Now take a long step to the left and note that the bars have gone to the right. Repeat 50 times.

PRACTICE NO. 2. Sit comfortably on a stool or a chair without resting the arms or back before a swing-stand. Place two flower pots or some other small objects 3 feet apart on each side about 6 feet away from the eyes. Move your body gently from side to side like a pendulum. When you move to the right, shift your body to the right side and glance at the right flower pot and *vice versa*. Note that the bars of the swing stand move in the opposite direction. Practice ten swings with the eyes open and ten swings with the eyes closed several times.

Then gradually decrease the distance in between the flower pots to 2 feet, 1 foot and six inches, while practising as before.

PRACTICE NO. 3. Arrange the swing stand and the flower pots as in No.2. Place an eye chart in between the flower pots. Move your body gently from side to side, shifting the sight from one flower pot to the other. Note that the bars move in the opposite direction and the chart moves in the direction of your body movement. Take care not to make any effort to see the chart.

PRACTICE NO. 4. Remove the flower pots. Place the chart at a distance from where you can see 3 or 4 lines of the chart. Arrange the swing-stand about 1 foot away from the eyes in such a way that you can see the chart through it.

Sit comfortably and sway the body. Move your sight on the white spaces in between the lines of letters, from one end to the other. Ignore reading of the letter. Note that the bars move in the opposite direction and the lines of the letters in the same direction. Repeat with the open and closed eyes for 10 minutes or more.

PRACTICE NO. 5. Same as No. 4. Move the sight on the white space below each letter and note that the few bars of the swing stand move in the opposite direction and the letter moves in the same direction. Body swing will be according to the width of the letter. Then swing with the closed eyes imagining the letter swinging. Then move on the white space below the next letter. Finish six or seven lines of the chart from 3 feet distance. Then gradually increase the distance of the chart to 10 or 20 feet by 3 or 4 inches each time.

EXAMPLE. The chart is at 3 feet distance and swing-stand at 1 foot distance from you, and you are able to read line 4th of the chart (5, C, G, O). Move your sight on the white space below 'R' of the second line without trying to see it. Note 'R' becomes darker and moves a little in the same direction. Do 5 times, then close the eyes and imagine it moving or swinging. Open the eyes and practise on 'B', and so on. Now suppose, you are able to practise on the 5th or 6th lines, increase the distance of the chart by 3 inches each time, practising on the 5th or 6th line. Other upper lines may be covered.

PRACTICE NO. 6. Place the test card at a distance where only the large letter 'C' at the top of the card can be distinguished. Stand with the feet about 9 inches apart and sway the body from side to side. When the body sways to the right, raise the left heel, put the weight of the body on the right leg, and look to the right of 'C' about 4 inches away. When the body sways to the left, raise the right heel, put the weight of the body on the left leg and look to the left of 'C', 4 inches away. Note that 'C' appears to be moving in the opposite direction. Now gradually shorten the sway and look to the right and left of 'C',4,3,1, half an inch away, noting all the time opposite movement of 'C'. The letter appears blacker when the movement is shorter. Repeat with the open and closed eyes.

PRACTICE NO. 7. Place the chart at a distance where you are able to read 5th or 6th line. Sit comfortably on a stool or a chair without resting the arms and back. Have a short movement of the body from side to side, and look to the right and left of each letter as in practice No 6. Note that each letter becomes blacker and appears to move in the opposite direction. Repeat the practice on each letter with open and closed eyes. The letter appears to pulsate. As the sight improves, increase the distance of the chart. Do not try to make the letters swing by effort. The swing should come of its own accord when the shifting is normal.

PRACTICE NO. 8.

(a) Place the Snellen Test Card at a distance at which it is seen best. In myopia this will be at the near point, a foot or less from the face. Look at a point about an inch or half above the top of the letter 'C'; then look at a point about an inch or half below the bottom part of the letter 'C'. While shifting the sight in this way note two things:

   1. The letter swings up and down.
   2. When the sight is near the top of the letter, the bottom part is seen worse; and when the sight is near the bottom, the top part is seen worse.

   Repeat about half a dozen times. If you feel any difficulty, rest the eyes, palm and try again.

(b) Now shift your sight to the top part of the letter noting that the bottom is seen worse. Then shift your sight from top to the bottom part of 'C' noting that the top is seen worse. While noting that each part is seen worse alternately, an illusion of swinging of the letter will be produced.

Now close the eye, and shift from the top to the bottom of the letter with the eyes closed. Repeat about three times with open eyes and three times with closed eyes.

Repeat the same procedure on the rest of the chart letters.

(c) Suppose you are able to produce the illusion of swinging of the letter both with the eyes closed and open. Now look at a blank wall. Close the eyes and keep up the mental swing of the letter.

Then regard the letter at a distance of five feet or more, and shift from the top to the bottom and *vice versa*. If successful, the letter will improve, and an illusion of swinging will be produced.

DIFFERENT KINDS OF SWINGS

Any of the following swinging exercises may be practised at the leisure times or during the course of practices on the chart to get relaxation.

1. LONG AND SHORT SWING

Stand with the feet about one foot apart, facing one side of the room, or the Snellen Test Card placed on the wall of the room. Lift the left heel a short distance from the floor while turning the shoulders, the head and the eyes to the right, until the line of shoulders is parallel with the wall. Now turn the body to the left after placing the left heel upon the floor and raising the right heel. Alternate, looking from the right wall to the left, being careful to move the head and the eyes with the movement of the shoulders. When practised easily, continuously, without effort and without paying any attention to moving objects, one soon feels that the long swing relaxes the tension of the muscles and the nerves. Then gradually shorten the long swing and practise the short swing. In the short swing the movement will be less than an inch.

Stationary objects appear to move with varying degrees of rapidity. Objects located almost directly in front of you appear to move with express train speed and are very much blurred. It is very important to make no attempt to see clearly objects which seem to be moving very rapidly.

The time taken in long swing should not be less than approximately one to two seconds each side. With many people the tendency is to gradually increase the speed and this is not helpful. Vigorous movements should be avoided.

2. SKY SWING

Stand facing the sky with the feet about one foot apart. Sway the body from side to side moving the sight on the sky without making any effort to see anything. Note that nearer objects appear to move in the opposite direction while farther objects appear to move in the same direction. At intervals of about two minutes close the eyes for a few seconds, sway and imagine the objects moving. One may stretch the arms to the sides like the wings of a bird and then sway. Practise for about ten minutes.

3. UNIVERSAL SWING

Under the cover of a cloth, move the thumb on the tip of your forefinger from side to side about one-quarter of an inch, and move your body gently with the thumb. Call 'one' when you move to the right, and 'two' when you move to the left. Close the eyes. Imagine your legs swinging in the direction opposite to your body. The floor on which the legs rest is also swinging. The walls of the room also swing when the floor swings. When one part of the building swings, one can imagine the whole building to be swinging. The ground on which the building stands is also swinging. When the ground swings, other buildings connected with it swing. One can imagine the whole city to be swinging, this continent and all other continents on the earth can be imagined swinging. In short, one can imagine not only that the whole world is moving, but also the universe including the sun, the moon and stars. If the direction is changed, strain results. To imagine the universal swing is easy, and some patients soon become able to do it with the eyes open.

4. CIRCULAR SWING

There is one objection to the universal swing, as at the end of the movement of the forefinger to the right or the left, one has a tendency to stop. This stoppage of the swing can be corrected by the practice of the circular swing, when all objects are imagined to move continuously in a circle. The circular swing can be realised with the eyes closed and differs from the other swings in this that the Snellen test card or other objects appear to move in a circular direction. In the circular swing, the head and the eyes are moved in a circular direction.

The circular swing realised by the movement of the Snellen Test Card or other objects appears to give complete relaxation of the mind and the eyes. Place your thumb on the tip of the forefinger and move it in a circle having a diameter of less than one-quarter of an inch. Move your body according to the movement of the thumb. While doing it notice that the thumb moves on the forefinger and the forefinger under the thumb, each moving in a direction opposite to that of the other. When done correctly, you will feel your whole body moving and everything about you will seem to move. Practise both with open and closed eyes.

5. MEMORY SWING

The memory swing relieves strain and tension as do the

long or the short swings. It is done with the eyes closed
while one imagines himself to be looking first over the right
shoulder and then over the left shoulder, while the head is
moved from side to side. The eyeballs may be seen through
the closed eyelids to move from side to side in the same
direction as the head is moved. When done properly, the
memory swing is just as efficient as the swing which is
practised with the eyes open, whether it is short or long.

The memory swing can be shortened by remembering the
swing of a small letter, a quarter of an inch or less, when
the eyes are closed.

The memory swing has given relief in many cases of imperfect sight from myopia, astigmatism and inflammations of
the outside of the eyeball as well as inflammations of the
inside of the eyeball. It is much easier than the swing
practised with the eyes open and secures a greater amount
of relaxation or rest than any swing. It may be practised in-
correctly, just as any swing may be done wrongly, and then
no benefit will be obtained.

6. VARIABLE SWING

Some patients feel difficulty in imagining the front objects
moving in the opposite direction. For such persons variable
swing is a great help.

The forefinger or a pencil is held about six inches in
front of the face, and a short distance to one side. By
looking straight ahead, without trying to see the finger, and
moving the head from side to side, the finger or the pencil
appears to move. This movement of the finger is greater
than the movement of objects at the distance. By practice,
patients become able to imagine not only the finger to be
moving, but also distant objects as well. Close the eyes and
imagine the movement of the finger while moving the head
and the eyes from side to side. Repeat with the eyes open
and closed.

7. FOREHEAD SWING

Place your fingers lightly on the forehead. Keep the eyes closed. Move your body and the head from side to side, but let the fingers be stationary at one place and allow the forehead to move freely beneath them. The fingers will appear to be moving in the the opposite direction while moving the head from side to side. The swing when practised in a right way proves very efficacious in relieving headache and pain in and around the eyeballs.

8. BABY SWING

Hold a baby and move it continuously in slow, short, easy curves, instead of moving the baby rapidly, irregularly, intermittently from side to side. This swing is very helpful for babies who suffer from restlessness or eye-strain.

9. FOOTBALL SWING

Move a ball with your foot. As the ball rolls forward the ground appears to move backwards. This is a very relaxing swing and a joyful game especially for elderly people.

10. ORBITAL SWING

Move the index finger of your hand in the form of an eclipse and follow its movement by moving the head and eyes together, first with eyes open, then with eyes closed. This swing is very useful in glaucoma cases in whom the eyeballs become static with a staring gait.

CHAPTER XI

ROUTINE TREATMENT

Routine treatment benefits a large number of patients; but to obtain the best results, it is necessary to modify the routine from time to time, or to make certain changes whenever improved methods of treatment are discovered. If a patient does not respond readily to a regular routine, it is an evidence that this treatment is not for him and that he requires a different form of relaxation treatment.

When a person presents himself for treatment, a record is made of his name, age, address, etc. The next procedure is to have the patient remove his glasses, if he is wearing them, and test the vision of each eye with the aid of the Snellen Test Card at fifteen feet or twenty feet. If none of the letters can be seen at this distance, the card is placed at ten feet, five feet or nearer and the vision tested at that distance. Then the sight is tested with glasses, on the Snellen Test Card at twenty feet. Then the near sight is tested on the Reading test type at six inches, nine inches or twelve inches, without and with glasses.

The eyes are then examined with the ophthalmoscope and retinoscope. (The ophthalmoscope is valuable in diagnosing cataract, opacities of the cornea and diseases of the interior of the eyeball. The retinoscope is used in diagnosing near-sightedness, far-sightedness and astigmatism.)

BLINKING: The patient is then directed to learn the correct way of keeping the upper eyelids and blinking.

SUN TREATMENT: The patient is then told to sit in the sun with the eyes closed, moving his body a short distance from side to side, and allowing the sun to shine directly on his closed eyelids. He is instructed to forget about his eyes, to think of something pleasant and let his mind drift from one pleasant thought to another. Application of honey or Resolvent 200 in the eyes just before sun treatment is a great help in many cases.

During summer when it is hot the patient usually keeps his feet in a tub full of cold water while facing the sun.

EYE WASH: After taking sun treatment the patient is directed to come to the shade and wash the eyes with cold water or triphala water or Ophthalmo Eye Wash.

PALMING: The patient then closes his eyes and palms for five to fifteen minutes. In palming, the patient closes both his eyes and covers them with the palms of both hands, in such a way so as to exclude all light. To palm successfully, he should make no effort to remember, imagine or see black. If black cannot be seen perfectly, the patient is told to let the mind drift from one pleasant thought to another. Some patients feel strain to remember something; they are asked to count 100 or 200 respirations while palming or are directed to keep the eyes closed and practise swinging before bars, universal swing or memory swing.

SHIFTING AND SWINGING: After the patient has rested his eyes by palming, he is directed to stand or sit before a swing stand and practise first long swing and then gradually shorten the long swing and practise the short swing. His attention is called to the fact that when his body, head and eyes move to the right, the bars of the swing-stand move to the left, and when he moves to the left, the bars appear to move to the right.

When the patient is able to practise the short swing, different practices of shifting and swinging exercises on the Snellen Test Card are demonstrated to him. Such exercises are needed to improve the distant vision or to prevent the staring habit.

CENTRAL FIXATION: When the patient is practising shifting and swinging before the Snellen Test Card, he is told to see one part of a letter, which he is regarding at a time, better than any other part, then quickly to shift his glance to another part, seeing that part best and other parts of the letter worse. The letter is seen much more readily in this way. The patient is reminded that the normal eye uses central fixation at all times.

SNELLEN EYE TEST CARD PRACTICE

You cannot see anything with perfect sight unless you have seen it before. When the eye looks at an unfamiliar object it always strains more or less to see that object, and an error of refraction is always produced. When the children look at unfamiliar writings or figures on the blackboard, distant maps, diagrams, or pictures, the retinoscope always shows that they are myopic, though their vision may be under other circumstances absolutely normal. The same thing happens when adults look at unfamiliar distant objects. When the eye regards a familiar object, however, the effect is quite otherwise. Not only can it be regarded without strain, but the strain of looking later at unfamiliar objects is lessened.

This fact furnishes us with a means of overcoming the mental strain to which the children are subjected by the modern educational system. It is impossible to see anything perfectly when the mind is under a strain, and if children become able to relax when looking at familiar objects, they become able, sometimes in an incredibly brief space of time, to maintain their relaxation when looking at unfamiliar objects. For this purpose practice on the Snellen Test Card is very useful.

1. Every home should have a Snellen Eye Test Card.

2. It is best to place a card permanently on the wall in good light.

3. Each member of the family or household should read the card every day.

4. It takes only a minute to test the sight with the card. If you spend five minutes in the morning for practising, it will be a great help during the day.

5. From above if you can only see down to the fourth line at fifteen feet distance, for example, notice that the last letter on that line is an "O", then close your eyes, cover them with the palms of the hands and remember the "O". If you will remember the picture of "O", it will help you to see the letter underneath the "O", which is "R".

6. If you stare at the letter "R", you will notice that all the letters on that line begin to blur. It is beneficial to close your eyes quickly after you see the "R", open the eyes, and shift to the first figure on that line which is 4. Then close your eyes and remember the 4, you will become able to read all the letters on that line by closing your eyes for each letter.

7. To see one letter of the card continuously, it is necessary to shift from one part of the letter to another. By alternately moving the eyes from one side of the letter to the other, it is possible to imagine the letter to be moving in the opposite direction to the movement of the eyes. This movement of the letter is called a swing. When it is slow, easy, short, about one quarter of an inch or less, maximum vision is obtained which continues as long as the swing continues.

8. While reading the card, blink on each letter and instead of fixing the sight on the black area, keep the sight on the white portion or look to the right and the left of the letter.

9. Practising with a familiar card is one of the quickest methods of curing myopia temporarily or permanently. The more perfectly the letters of the card are remembered or imagined, the more completely is the myopia relieved.

10. In cases of nervous patients or children, point to the first letter of each line by putting your finger half an inch below each letter and tell the patient to look in the direction of the finger tip and not at the letter.

11. Stand and sway, or sit in a comfortable chair, and rest your legs and feet on a stool which is as high as the seat of your chair. Read the card lazily, and comfortably

and gently blink as you read. Read the test card with your better eye and then palm. Read the test card with your worse eye and then palm. Read the test card with both eyes together and then palm. Practise with the pot-hooks chart as follows: Name or indicate with the hand the direction in which the letter points. Copy the chart, using white paper and black pencil. Read it with the weaker eye covering the other with a pad.

12. When difficulty is experienced in reading certain letters on the chart, one or more of the following methods may be tried:

(a) Palm, then remove the hands and swing; read the chart, close the eyes after reading each letter.

(b) Read the fine print as close to the eyes as possible, avoiding strain, and then read the chart.

(c) Close the eyes for a few seconds, and look at the left side of the letter, report its appearance, repeat with the right side of the letter, then read the letter.

(d) Walk up to the chart, read the letter. Return to the former position and read it.

13. Note from the diagrams how to keep your eye covered while reading the chart.

14. Keep a record of each test in order to note your progress from day to day.

TEST TYPE

READING FINE PRINT

1. The reading of large types in preference to finer print is a bad habit. It requires more of an effort to see a large letter than a small letter, strange as it may seem. When you look at the big "C" on the Snellen Test Card, you

don't see it all at once. You have to look at one part
best. Some people think they see the whole of it at the
same time, but that is not the case. Their eyes shift from
one point to another unconsciously.

2. Blink frequently, at least at the beginning and at the
end of each line of ordinary type.

3. Do not look at the letters, but at the white spaces
between them, and imagine them whiter than the margin.
It is a general belief that when we read, we are looking
at the letters. When one reads with the perfect sight, one
does not look at the letters, but at the white spaces between the lines and imagines the white centres of the letters to be whiter than they really are. Look directly at a
small letter of the fine print that can be read and concentrate your mind and eyes on one part of the letter. You
soon feel an effort or strain and the vision is always
lowered. If the vision is not lowered, that means that you
are unable to keep your attention fixed on the same part
of a small letter for a continuous length of time. When
one plans to look at the white spaces and, while trying to
read something, feels discomfort or pain, it means that the
eyes are not directed on the white spaces as the reader
may imagine.

4. Move the head a little from side to side or gently
sway the body forward and backward as sometimes children
do in the schools while reading. Keeping the head and the
eyes stationary causes strain and lowers the vision.

5. If your eyes feel strained and do not want to read
more, stop and palm for a few minutes. You will notice
that where it looked all blurred before, it will appear clear
and distinct now.

6. Read the fine print as close to the eyes as possible
both morning and evening, in good light as well as in dim
light, without or with glasses. It will keep your near sight
strong and prevent eye troubles that generally appear in old
age.

7. Reading the familiar types is always more beneficial than an unfamiliar one.

To improve reading use a card hole.

8. Before practising on the reading test type, have sun treatment and it will help you a great deal. The letters, which you were quite unable to read, will become distinct and clear. Frequent practices will make that improvement permanent. Hold a card of fine print (Reading test type) about ten inches from the eyes. Read as much as you can. Now face the sun with closed eyelids for five minutes or more. Come to your former seat, sit comfortably and cover the eyes with the palms of your hands for two minutes or more. Then read the test type while blinking freqently. You will notice a decided improvement in your sight.

FINE PRINT: The patient is directed to practise with the fine print on the Fundamental card or with the photo print in the following way: the card is held at first at the distance from his eyes at which he sees best. He is told not to look directly at the letters but just at the white spaces between the lines of print and imagine that they are perfectly white — whiter than the margin. He is asked if he can imagine that there is a thin white line beneath each line of letters and that it is whiter than the rest of the white spaces between the lines. When this line is imagined perfectly white, the letters are read without effort or strain. The patient is told to blink as he shifts from one end of the line to the other, to occasionally look away and to close his eyes frequently for half a minute or so to rest them.

By practising in this way, letters which could not be seen before appear black and distinct. As one's ability to read is improved, the card is brought closer in hypermetropic or old age patients, or the distance of the card is increased in myopic cases. The patient is told that the reading of fine print and photo print is helpful in producing relaxation. Reading fine print in good light and candle light proves extremely beneficial.

INSTRUCTIONS FOR HOME TREATMENT: —

1. After waking up from the sleep, in the morning practise the long swing 100 times or run in a circle or palm
for 5 minutes.
2. At the time of dressing, remember blinking and sway
gently.
3. While walking imagine side objects or the ground
moving backwards.
4. Before retiring to bed practise palming or long swing
with the memory of a black dot or count 100 to 200 respirations.
5. Read Fine Print in candle light.

BENEFIT TO CHILDREN AND ADULTS

Every family should obtain a Snellen Test Card and
place it on the wall of some room where it can be seen
and read every day by all the members of the family. Not
only does the daily reading of the card help to keep up
the visual acuity in children, but it is a benefit to the eyes
of adults as well.

It is a well-known fact that when most people arrive at
the age of forty or fifty years, they find that their vision
for reading or sewing is lowered. These people believe that
they must put on glasses to prevent eye-strain, cataract,
glaucoma, etc. Daily practice with the Snellen Test Card
together with the reading of fine print close to the eyes
will overcome their difficulty. Reading fine print close to
the eyes, contrary to the usually accepted opinion of many
ophthalmologists, is a benefit to the eyes of both children
and adults.

It has been repeatedly demonstrated, however, that fine
print cannot be read clearly or easily when an effort is

made. When the eyes look directly at the letters, an effort is required, while looking at the white spaces between the lines gives the needed rest, and by practice in this way, one can become able to see the letters clearly, without looking directly at them. When a patient looks at the white spaces between the lines of ordinary book type, he can read for hours and no fatigue, pain or discomfort is felt. When discomfort and pain in the eyes is felt while reading, it is because the patient is looking directly at the letters.

No Glasses For Quick Results

Generally persons who have never worn glasses are more easily cured than those who have, and glasses should be discarded at the beginning of the treatment. It is not always an easy thing to do, but it is the best for the patient. During the treatment when the glasses are worn temporarily, even for a short time, the vision sometimes becomes worse and in most cases a relapse is produced. When the patient has to continue his work during the treatment and cannot do so without glasses, their use may be permitted for a time, and the power of the glasses can be reduced gradually, but this always delays the cure.

Some people complain that no glasses fit their eyes permanently. These cases are benefited by discarding their glasses for a longer or shorter period while being treated.

The time required to effect a permanent cure varies greatly with different individuals. In some cases fifteen minutes are sufficient, and I believe the time is coming when it will be possible to cure every one quickly. It is only a question of accumulating more facts, and presenting these facts in such a way that the patient can grasp them quickly. In most cases, the treatment must be continued for a few minutes every day to prevent relapse. When a cure is complete, it is always permanent. Even in such cases, the treatment can be continued with benefit. It is not al-

ways easy to treat the more severe cases. When the patient
has been under a strain for a length of time, it is sometimes difficult to relieve the strain permanently in a short
time. Patients vary in their response to treatment. While
some obtain permanent relief within a short time, others
find it necessary to place themselves under the treatment
for a longer period.

Daily practice of the art of vision is also necessary to
prevent those lapses to which every eye is liable no matter how good its sight ordinarily may be. The daily reading of small, distant, familiar letters will do much to lessen
the tendency to strain when disturbing circumstances arise.

Persons of all ages have been benefited by Bates' methods of relaxation; but children under twelve years of age
respond very quickly.

CORRESPONDENCE TREATMENT

Many letters are received from people in various parts
of India who find it impossible to come to my office and
also believe that something might be done for them by
correspondence treatment. I do not advocate correspondence
treatment as a general rule, as the results are uncertain.
There is always the possibility that the patient will not
practise correctly the things which he is told to do. If the
patient had had one treatment at my office, it is possible
to treat the patient more intelligently through correspondence. When this book is read carefully, those things which
are not understood may be cleared up by intelligent questions which I am always ready to answer. I do not consider this regular correspondence treatment very useful.

No doubt, in certain cases very remarkable results have
been obtained by correspondence treatment. A boy wearing glasses of -4.0 got instructions by correspondence and
in a week's time he made his eyesight normal at different
distances. Many other patients suffering from different sorts

of eye defects have also been benefited by correspondence treatment, but many a time it has been noted that cases which did not improve by correspondence were soon benefited after visiting my clinic.

WRONG BELIEFS

1. GLASSES PREVENT AND CURE EYE DEFECTS:

While prescribing glasses patients are made to believe that the use of glasses will prevent the eye defect or check further deterioration; but within a short time they experience that in spite of the use of glasses according to the prescription the sight has gone worse. In 90% of the cases who depend on the use of the glasses, the defect in eyesight goes on increasing and the glasses are frequently changed.

A patient who adopts palming treatment and discards glasses temporarily or permanently is frequently cautioned by the doctors and others that the eyes would get strain without glasses. Such persons may be asked the following questions.

(a) What are the symptoms if the eye strains without glasses?

(b) If the symptoms of eye strain are not present without glasses, then why should not glasses be discarded to improve the eyesight?

(c) If one does not feel comfortable with glasses or if the number of glasses goes on increasing in spite of their constant use, then, is that not the sign of eye strain?

2. EYESIGHT DETERIORATES AS THE AGE ADVANCES:

The belief that the eyesight deteriorates as the age advances specially when one passes fortieth year is wrong.

The eyes are one of the sense organs. When other sense organs like ear, nose, etc., do not become defective or old as the age advances, then, why should the eye? Could Nature leave the organ of sight defectively developed when most of the functions of life depended on the eye? Every one can keep up good eyesight throughout life like other senses by the practice of relaxation methods for a few minutes. If persons, who find themselves getting presbyopic or who have arrived at presbyopic age, would instead of resorting to glasses, practise reading the finest print they can find, the idea that the eyesight declines as a result of growing old would die a natural death.

3. READING OF FINE PRINT IS BAD FOR THE EYES:

It is a general belief that reading of fine print is harmful to the eyes. In fact FINE PRINT IS A BENEFIT TO THE EYES WHILE LARGE PRINT IS A MENACE. Reading of fine print, when it can be done without discomfort, has invariably proved to be beneficial, and dimmer the light in which it can be read and closer to the eyes it can be held, the greater the benefit. The reason is that fine print cannot be read in a dim light and close to the eyes unless the eyes are relaxed, whereas large print can be read in a good light and at ordinary reading distance although the eyes may be under a strain. When fine print can be read under adverse conditions, the reading of ordinary print under ordinary conditions is improved vastly. One should read fine print daily in good light and in candle light.

CHAPTER XII

EYESIGHT OF SCHOOL CHILDREN

Imperfect sight is found in the eyes of most school children of India and other countries. It is a truth that nearly all the cases of imperfect sight in school children are acquired after they enter the school. Their eyes are normal when they begin their school life. After a few years, most of them acquire imperfect sight, the average being about eighty per cent. Of these, nearly all have acquired far-sightedness and astigmatism. At the age of ten or twelve, near-sightedness appears, and far-sightedness in children becomes less. It is a general belief that strain to see at the near point causes short-sightedness (myopia); but, in the preceding chapter, it has been clearly shown that a strain at the near point always produces far-sightedness (hypermetropia). To check the strain at the near point, the authorities laid down different rules as to the size of types to be used in school books, amount and arrangement of light, construction of desks, etc. The result of these preventing measures was disappointing and the prevalence of myopia did not stop.

The truth is that the strain to see at a distance causes near-sightedness or myopia. Why do some children strain at the distance and gain myopia while others do not strain at all and have perfect sight? Experience shows that all persons are not created equal to one another. Some children come to know that strain lowers the vision, but they go on straining, because they do not know what else to do.

Children are great imitators. They learn to walk by watching others walk. They learn to talk and play from the examples of other children. Similarly, they learn to strain the eyes from their teachers, parents, friends and others. Parents and teachers, who use glasses and strain their eyes affect the mind of the children. Some children suffer so

much from headache and other troubles when attending
school that they easily acquire strain from others. The
following also affect the eyesight: —

1. Punishment either physical or mental.
2. Temperament of the people with whom the child comes
   into contact.
3. Nervousness of the children.
4. Uninteresting subjects.

CURE: 1. Teachers should learn how to have normal sight
without glasses.

2. Teachers should explain to the students how to avoid
strain by blinking, palming and swinging.

3. Daily practice on the Snellen Test Card for five minutes
in the school (see the scheme of preventing myopia in
schools).

4. Once a week, eye education should be given to the
children. It is an encouraging fact that children, soon after
they are cured of their defects in eyesight without the aid
of glasses, have a great desire to help others and the more
they try to help others, the greater the benefit to themselves.

5. Before you make up your mind to compel a child to
use glasses, ask the child to practise relaxation method.

PREVENTION OF MYOPIA IN SCHOOLS

Place the Snellen Test Card upon the wall of each class-
room. Every day, the children should read silently the
smallest letters they can see from their seats, with both eyes
together and then with each eye separately, the other eye
being covered with the palm of the hand, avoiding any
pressure upon the eyeball.

Appoint a period of five minutes for it in the beginning
of school work. It should be the duty of the teachers to
note that all children read the test card with blinking. The
practice of five minutes daily is sufficient to improve the
sight of all children in one week and to cure defective eye-

sight after some time.

Children with markedly defective vision should be encouraged to read the chart more frequently and practise palming at home. Children wearing glasses should not be interfered with, as they are supposed to be under the care of physicians and the practice will do them little or no good while the glasses are worn.

Though not necessary, it is of a great advantage to have records made of each pupil at the time when the method is introduced, and thereafter at convenient intervals annually or more frequently. This may be done by the teachers. The records should include the name and the age of the pupil, the vision of each eye tested, and the date.

How to test the Vision? Keep the Snellen Chart at twenty feet distance from the student and ask him to read the chart with each eye separately, keeping the other eye covered by the palm of the hand. Write the result in the form of a fraction with the distance at which the line of letters is read as the numerator and the distance at which the line ought to be read as the denominator. The figures above the line of letters on the test card indicate the distance at which these letters should be read by persons with normal sight. Suppose, Mr. Mohanram, aged fifteen reads at 20 feet distance the fifty feet line with the right eye and at ten feet distance the 200 feet line with the left eye, then write: —

Date	Name	Age	1st test		Date	2nd tets		Date	3rd test	
			R. E.	L. E.		R. E.	L. E.		R. E.	L. E.
1.9.'40	Mr. Mohanram	15	$\frac{20}{50}$	$\frac{10}{200}$	1.10.'40	$\frac{20}{40}$	$\frac{20}{100}$	12.12.'40	$\frac{20}{20}$	$\frac{20}{50}$

A certain amount of supervision is absolutely necessary. At least once a year, one who understands the methods should visit each class-room for the purpose of helping and encouraging the teachers to continue the use of the methods rightly and making some kind of report to the proper authorities. It is not necessary that the supervisor, the teacher or the children should understand anything about the physiology of the eye. This scheme will save many students from becoming myopic. Try it in the schools at least for a year and keep the record. Compare it with the results of the previous year; you will be convinced of the fact.

Then why should our children be compelled to suffer any more and wear glasses for want of this simple measure of relief? Lots of money are spent in spectacles every year. This system costs practically nothing. Simply there is the need of a Snellen Test Card in each class-room. No one would venture to suggest that this scheme could possibly do any harm. Why, then, should there be any delay about introducing it into schools?

This plan for eyesight conservation was followed by the institutions of Khurja, (U.P.). First, I delivered lectures on the subject and visited each class-room and explained the methods clearly. Great care was taken to make the reports accurate. The tests were made by the class-room teachers. In all 820 eyes were examined and 249 were recorded defective at the beginning of the session. During the year, the pupils were encouraged merely to read the Snellen Test Card daily. At the close of the year again, the eyes of the same students were examined and 99 out of 249 defective eyes had attained normal vision, while 85 showed improvement.

Principal Chunilal Majumdar of Khurja writes:

"Dr. Raghubir Sharan Agarwal delivered lectures in my college on the prevention of myopia. The scheme was explained with facts and I introduced it in the classes. I took the results of the vision of students before beginning the scheme. I set apart a period of about five minutes for the students to have a daily practice. After six months, I secured the results again and found a marvellous progress and improvement in the cases of defective vision."

Q. What are the benefits of this chart reading scheme?

A. 1. Improvement in eyesight.

2. Headaches or other discomforts are relieved or prevented.

3. Ability to study is improved.

4. Mental faculties are improved.

5. Truancy becomes less.

6. Mischievous and restless boys become good pupils.

Q. If strain at distant objects causes myopia then why is it more prevalent in schools and colleges where the students devote most of the time to reading?

A. When the eye accommodates itself for reading, the eyeball is elongated. Excessive accommodation produces a permanent elongation of the eyeball when the eye strains to see distant objects.

Q. Is it not that when the child reads the same chart daily, he remembers it by heart and then reading of the same chart will not be beneficial?

A. Daily reading of the familiar chart is very beneficial. The memory of the letters help the children to relax themselves, and they can read more lines of the chart.

Q. What is the most helpful exercise for children?

A. Palming is generally most helpful.

A short narrative describing the benefits derived from palming by one of the schoolboys benefited:

1. Palming is one of the works that has helped me in room six. While writing a story it would help me in my imagination. When I first came to room six Arithmetic was very hard for me to learn, but now it is as easy as punk.

2. About a month ago I told my sister to start palming. She has glasses and I would not like her to have them any longer. She has started, and it seems likely she will soon

have eyes that will not need glasses.

3. Palming and the Snellen Card did me a great deal of good. It gave me more strength in my imagination, and I can do my work much better everyday. I am not sorry in knowing how to palm, because in the beginning I did not like to put my hands over my eyes.

4. I told my mother to palm; it would help her, but she did not believe me. One day I said, "Mother, palm." She said, "All right." Finally a week later she could see clearly. She said, "I am glad I did what you told me."

5. Palming is a wonderful treatment for the eyes. It has done much during one and a half years. It has strengthened our imagination, rested our eyes, and kept them from wearing glasses.

6. We have a palming lesson four times a day. While we are palming we have a little music to think of something pleasant. It has cured headache in many of us. It is spreading everywhere and we see lots of people doing it now.

7. It is very good for me. It settled my mind. I do not get so excited, and can add my columns easier. I can palm, if I get nervous.

VISUAL EDUCATION

Poor eyesight is admitted to be the cause of retardation at school. In many cases defective vision is the result of an abnormal condition of the mind, the mind is under a strain, and when the mind is under strain the process of education cannot be conducted successfully. By putting glasses on the child we may make the child to see better but we are not able to relieve the strain which underlies the imperfect functioning. The result is that the power of glasses goes on increasing more and more.

When the mind is under strain, memory is the first to be affected. The extraordinary memory and keenness of vision of primitive people was due to the mind being at rest. When one is not interested, one's mind is not under control, and without mental control one can neither learn nor see. A teacher reported that one of her pupils used to sit doing nothing all day long and apparently was not interested in any thing. After reading the eye testing card daily his sight improved, he became anxious to learn, and speedily developed into one of the best students of the class. In other words his eyes and mind became normal together.

Unfamiliar objects always cause strain on the minds of the children. Hence children learning to read, write, draw, or sew often suffer from defective vision and discomforts of the eyes and head. Headache is a frequent occurence. This is due to the unfamiliarity of the lines or objects with which the children are working. Such children can be greatly helped by reading fine print and eye chart daily with gentle blinking. The art of seeing pictures proves wonderfully helpful in the improvement of eyesight. Games which keep the children in motion become an aid to eyesight.

ART OF SEEING

Almost every eye specialist of the world believes that for the refractive errors as myopia and hypermetropia there is not only no cure, practically no preventive also. From such a belief any rational mind will conclude that science is yet in a very imperfect stage. What some writers on Ophthalmology wrote two hundred years back about the incurability of visual defects, is continuing as a dogma even today, in the days of advanced science. We are so much hypnotised by the assertions of the old authorities that we do not care to make any experiment or do some research on the subject. And if anyone comes forward to say that cases of visual defects could be improved without glasses, we begin to doubt and without any study discard his explanation. Such is the condition of our mind which is supposed to be scientific. A scientific mind is always open to admit a truth or a fact.

The old writers on Ophthalmology did not consider that the mental strain could play an important part in the formation of visual defects, hence they isolated the eye while determining the cause and treatment. To rectify the effect of errors of refraction they prescribed glasses. But very little has ever been claimed about their usefulness except that these contrivances neutralize the effects of the various conditions for which they are prescribed, as a crutch enables a lame man to walk.

All along it has been my experience that mental relaxation is the key to success in life, in education and treatment of patients. Under the present conditions of life man's mind is under a severe strain, hence all sorts of visual defects are taking place and we are curing these visual defects through eye education and mental relaxation very successfully.

The School for Perfect Eyesight has developed a new technique called the 'art of seeing' for the cure of visual defects. Itisri and Lipi, two Oriya girls, 10-year old, studying in Sri Aurobindo International Centre of Education, Pondicherry had developed a condition of semi-blindness (Amblyopia). Their vision was found defective both for distance and near without any apparent cause and the glasses did not help them to see better. The teacher told us that the defective condition had developed after joining the school class. It is important to note that when children begin to learn unfamiliar things, letters or a language, they usually suffer from little or more of eye strain and mental strain due to the unfamiliarity of the lines and figures and letters. It is at this stage that visual defects usually start. And if children can be taught a few simple methods of eye education their defects will soon fade away and they will enjoy perfect eyesight. Let me tell you how these two semi-blind girls were cured in fifteen minutes by the art of seeing "view cards and pictures."

I taught these girls the art of seeing pictures with the mind completely relaxed. I gave a view card depicting a colourful picture of Taj Mahal to them. Soon the flatness began to disappear and the three-dimensional character of the picture was clearly perceived by the girls. With the mind relaxed, the picture appeared so beautiful to the eyes that their minds got deeply absorbed in seeing the Taj. They exclaimed, Lovely! Beautiful! the details of the picture were appearing sharply, they were observing that their vision was getting improved. Then when they were asked to read the Snellen Eye Testing Chart from 10ft and 20ft. they could easily read the normal line after a few attempts. They could also read the fine print which was impossible before. Since then they are maintaining permanent improvement. Formerly defective vision of this nature in children was cured in about two weeks but now by the art of seeing it was corrected in 15 minutes. Further experiments have proved that this exercise of mind and eyes proves very helpful in the improvement of eyesight in almost all cases who can successfully do it. Of course, in the case of older persons it takes longer time to effect a cure due to lack of good imagination. A teacher of our Centre of Education whose left eye had been blind since childhood, regained normal eyesight within two months with regular eye exercises for about two hours a day.

The School for Perfect Eyesight has developed a sort of synthesis of all the systems for practical working to achieve wonderful results. Our aim is to create a new type of doctor whose knowledge will be based on such a synthesis, who will be guided by the higher intelligence, who will be more concerned with health than with pathology.

DISCOVERY OF THE ART OF SEEING: Our girl patient Lipi about whom I have mentioned above complained about her bad eyesight both for distance and near, she often experienced pain and headache while reading. When tested on the Snellen Test Card, she could hardly read four lines from 10ft. distance and she could not read small print. The retinoscope indicated that she was having hypermetropic astigmatism. She was put on different eye exercises but the results were not quite satisfactory. What to do? In the meantime I had received a view card of Angel Bridge from a Russian friend, I found myself absorbed in seeing its beauty, very soon I found that the bridge appeared as if a reality in a three-dimensional character. Next day a friend presented a colourful picture of Taj Mahal Agra and I found this view card of Taj Mahal more charming and beautiful, very relaxing to the mind. Anything which relaxes the mind is a benefit to the eyesight. So I gave a picture of Taj Mahal to this girl patient. She was asked to look at the people right in front and at those who were on the floor of Taj Mahal as if they were a mile away, very far. By alternate shifting of sight she could feel the distance between the people in front and the Taj Mahal. Taj Mahal appeared as if a real monument before her. Instantly the girl observed that the sun had also come there as if from no where and was shining brilliantly on the golden dresses of the girls in the photograph. Suddenly she cried out, "Ah, it is really beautiful." She saw the depth in the windows of the Taj Mahal. The shadows of the front walls of the Taj falling on the walls behind added to its three-dimensional appearance. The four minars, the conical trees, the water canal and the carpet of green grass, all appeared quite real to her. The mind got hypnotised to see everything in its true perspective, as if Taj was visible with its length, breadth and height. The people in front seemed to be walking in reality. Their feet would rise and fall in front. The coloured saree of the lady became hundred-fold beautiful and magnificent with all its sober designs. When the mind got completely relaxed, the visual cells of the retina began to function with their full capacity.

Amazingly when Lipi looked at the Snellen Test Card, she could read two lines more and ultimately within fifteen minutes her sight was normal both for distance and near. My assistant got so much excited that he took the retinoscope to test her sight in the dark room and it was found that there was no more astigmatism. Both eyes became normal without the least sign of error of refraction.

To see whether she could retain the relaxation while looking at an unfamiliar object, I placed a different Snellen Test Card before her, she could read the new chart also from 10ft. and 20ft. showing that her vision was perfectly all right.

A few days later Itisri came with almost same trouble and same defective vision. The new technique was applied on her with the same success. She too was all right in 15 minutes. We then tried this new exercise of art of seeing on other patients of all ages and all defects and found it quite effective when done properly. But for children it is a boon which brings instantaneous relief.

CHAPTER XIII

DIET

It is not necessary that a person taking unbalanced diet should suffer from defective eyesight, or that a person taking good nourishing and balanced diet should not suffer from defective eyesight because the cause of defective eyesight is staring and not diet. Many persons having a good diet suffer from high errors of refraction, while many persons having an unbalanced diet have good eyesight. But it does not mean that one should avoid the rules of diet. Good diet is a help to keep the body and mind healthy and the relaxation is helped indirectly. Persons who have the habit of making an effort to see and at the same time suffer from indigestion or constipation due to unbalanced diet suffer more and in some cases a serious condition of the eye develops. A good diet is a great help in the treatment of many inflammatory and chronic diseases of the eye.

The body requires certain articles, and each of them in a certain quantity, for its proper nourishment. Substitution of one article by another can be done within only certain well-defined limits. If the change is made with indiscretion, ill-health is sure to follow. Granted that the proper food is taken, you will help it by a proper mastication, taking it in a suitable quantity, according to the digestive power, and at sufficient intervals. I will give the general principles and every one can easily select the best food suited to his constitution, by trying it for himself.

The chemical composition of blood and lymph depends upon the chemical composition of food and drink, and upon the normal or abnormal condition of the digestive organs. The system of dietetics is based upon the composition of milk, which is the only perfect natural food combination in existence. In eye diseases, a vegetarian diet is prefered, and the change from a meat diet to a non-meat diet is of a great benefit in the treatment of chronic eye diseases as retinitis, choroiditis, optic atrophy, high myopia, glaucoma, iritis, etc.

In the accompanying table, entitled "Dietetics in a Nutshell", we have divided all food materials into five groups.

As a general rule, let one half of your food consist of Group V, and the other half of a mixture of the first four groups.

The following is a fair list of wholesome foods.

DAIRY PRODUCTS: Milk, buttermilk, skimmed milk, cream, butter, fresh cottage cheese, curd. Cows' milk is rich in vitamin A, and proves very useful in retinal and choroidal diseases.

EGGS: Either raw, soft-boiled or poached, not fried or hard-boiled. One egg a day is sufficient. White of egg is much easier to digest than the yolk. Therefore, the white should only be used in cases having a weak digestion.

HONEY: A very valuable food and a natural laxative, and is one of the best forms of sugar. It should not be mixed in hot water or hot things.

CEREAL FOODS: Rice, wheat, barley, gram, etc., are good when properly combined with fruits and vegetables and with dairy products. Use preferably the whole grain preparations. Avoid the use of white bread or any other white flour products, especially pastry. Barley flour is a very good food in chronic retinal diseases. It may be taken alone or mixed with wheat flour.

A good substitute for bread is the following: Whole wheat preparation: Smash wheat into pieces (called Dalia) and soak in cold water for about one hour and boil for about two hours. Eat with honey and milk. Add raisins. This dish is very nutritious and one of the finest laxatives and easily digestible foods. Oats porridge may be substituted.

DIETETICS IN A NUTSHELL

Food classes.	Functions in Vital Processes.	Food in which the elements of the respective groups predominate.
GROUP I — CARBOHYDRATES Starches and Dextrines.	Producers of Heat and Energy.	CEREALS: The inner, white parts of wheat, corn, oats, barley and rice. VEGETABLES: Potatoes, roots, pumpkins. FRUITS: Bananas. NUTS: Chestnuts.
GROUP II — CARBOHYDRATES Sugars.	Producers of Heat and Energy.	VEGETABLES: Melons, beets. FRUITS: Bananas, dates, figs, grapes, raisins. DAIRY PRODUCTS: Milk. NATURAL SUGARS: Honey. COMMERCIAL SUGARS: White sugar, syrup, glucose, candy. NUTS: Cocoanuts.
GROUP III — HYDROCARBONS Fats and Oils.	Producers of Heat and Energy.	FRUITS: Olives. DAIRY PRODUCTS: Cream, butter, cheese. NUTS: Almonds, walnuts, cocoanuts, peanuts, etc. COMMERCIAL FATS: Olive oil, vegetable-cooking oil. The yolks of eggs.

Group		Producers / Function	Foods
GROUP IV — ORGANIC PROTEINS	Albumen (white of egg) Gluten (grains) Myosin (Lean meat).	Producers of Heat and Energy; Building and Repair Materials for Cells and Tissues.	CEREALS: The outer, dark parts of wheat, corn, oats; barley and rice. VEGETABLES: Peas, beans, lentils, mushrooms. NUTS: Cocoanuts, chestnuts, peanuts, walnuts, etc. DAIRY PRODUCTS: Milk cheese. MEATS: Muscular parts of animals, fish and fowls.
GROUP V — ORGANIC MINERALS — MINERALS	Organic Mineral Elements.	Eliminators; Blood, Bone and Nerve Builders; Laxatives; Cholagogues, Producers of Electro-Magnetic Energies.	CEREALS: The husk and outer dark layers of grains and rice. VEGETABLES: Lettuce, spinach, cabbage, green peppers, water-cress, celery, onions, cauliflower, tomatoes, string-beans, fresh peas, cucumbers, radishes, beets, carrots, turnips, pumpkins, squashes. FRUITS: Apples, pears, peaches, oranges, lemons, grapefruit, plums, prunes, apricots, cherries, olives, berries, mangoes. DAIRY PRODUCTS: Milk, butter-milk, skimmed milk. NUTS: Cocoanuts.

VEGETABLES: Peas and beans in the green state are good vegetables. Lettuce, spinach, cabbage, watercress, celery, parsley, Brussels-sprouts rank highest in organic mineral salts. Next to these come tomatoes, cucumbers, green peppers, radishes, onions, asparagus, cauliflower, horse radish, pumpkins, squashes and melons. Strong spices and condiments should be avoided in cooking vegetables. Cook vegetables as long as is required to make them soft enough for easy mastication. Do not throw away a drop of water in which vegetables have been cooked.

FRUIT AND BERRIES: Lemons, grapefruits, oranges, mangoes, apples, plums, pears, peaches, apricots and cherries are very beneficial.

DRIED FRUITS: Prunes, dates, figs and raisins.

Bananas differ from the juicy fruits. They consist almost entirely of starches, dextrines and sugars. They should be used sparingly by people suffering from intestinal indigestion. They are an excellent food, especially for children.

Fruits and vegetables may be mixed in the same meal.

First eat hard things as bread, then softer things as rice etc., liquids in the last as milk, soups.

VITAMIN A — Clinical and experimental evidence indicates that Vitamin A is essential for the normal function of the retina and its use is helpful in myopia, retinal and choroidal diseases.

Vitamin A is present in cow's milk, carrot, cod-liver oil, butter, pumpkin, spinach, tomatoe, pineapple, peas, fresh fish. Abidol, Nestrovit and *Tirphala Ghrita* are good medicines containing Vitamin A.

The human body is made up of acid and alkaline constituents (*Pitta and Kapha*). In order to have the normal conditions and functions of tissues and organs, both must be present in the right proportions. Groups No. I, II, III and IV are generally acid forming and No. V alkaline forming. When the intake of acid forming diet becomes excessive or there is defective elimination of waste material through faeces, urine and perspiration, the amount of acid is increased beyond a certain limit. The blood loses its power to dissolve it, and it forms a sticky, glue-like, "colloid" substance, which occludes or blocks up the minute blood vessels (capillaries), so that the blood cannot pass readily from the arterial system into the venous circulation. This interference with the normal circulation and distribution of the blood interferes with the normal functions of the eye. Diseases of retina and choroid are generally due to defective circulation of blood through the capillaries.

QUANTITY OF FOOD — No hard and fast general rule can be laid down. You yourself are the best judge. When you are satisfied, but not too full, stop. Fasting for one day every week proves very useful. One may clear the bowels by an enema once a week.

IMPORTANCE OF WATER — Water may be avoided during a meal, because it hinders the secretion of saliva and gastric juice. Besides any quantity of the juices secreted will be diluted and made weaker. A few sips may be taken if at all necessary.

Water should be taken between the meals. If you drink a glass of water in the morning and one at the time of going to bed, it helps in the movements of the bowels, especially if the water is warm. Three hours after meals or one hour before meals is a good interval to drink. But do not drink too much even then; otherwise you will be waterlogged and water-logging is very harmful.

If you get over-thirsty, it means that your inside is not correct and you require a short fast of a day or two and an enema of simple warm water and lemon juice or stomach-intestine wash; the details may be studied from 'Secrets of Indian Medicine'.

EXERCISE

Exercise is very important. The best exercise for every one is walking. About four or five miles a day is quite sufficient. Gardening is also very good. One can have some jerking exercises for 10 or 15 minutes. When walking or taking any other exercise, take deep breaths at intervals. This will open all the smallest air cells in the lungs which play an important part in purifying the blood. For exercise, you should generally go to open air and sunshine, which are very beneficial to health. Stop exercise when feeling just tired. Let the muscles work smoothly.

While performing any exercise, take care of the position of the eye lids. Do not open the eyes widely. Many athletes take their exercises before a mirror. They are told to look at the muscle which they are exercising in order to feel that it is growing in bulk and strength. This leads them to fix their gaze on the particular muscle in the mirror; blinking is stopped. As the exercise of that muscle may last many minutes, it leads to staring which affects the eyes adversely.

What should be done then? Blinking should not be stopped and the sight should continually shift from one part of the muscle to another part. Almost all the exercises involve the movement of the body or parts of it, either up and down or backwards and forwards. The general tendency is to leave the eyes staring in the front while the body moves, and this attitude is wrong. Shift your sight according to the movement of the body. At every movement of your body, imagine that the stationary objects are moving in the opposite direction. If you move forward as in the exercise *Dand*, the front objects and the ground should be imagined to be moving backward, and when you move backward, the objects should be imagined to be moving forward. With the exercise *Baithak*, the objects seem to be jumping up and down.

WALKING: While walking, running or riding, etc., imagine that the ground and side objects move backwards.

Many people have complained that after walking a short distance slowly, easily and without any special effort, they become nervous, tired and their eyes feel the symptoms and consequences of a strain. When they were taught the correct way to use their eyes while walking, the symptoms of a fatigue or strain disappeared.

The fact can be demonstrated with the aid of a straight line on the floor or the seam in the carpet.

Stand with the right foot to the right of the line and the left foot to the left of the line. Now put your right foot forward and look to the left of the line. Then put your left foot forward and look to the right of the line. Note that it is difficult to do this longer than a few seconds without discomfort, pain, headache, dizziness or nausea.

Now, practise the right method of walking and using the eyes. When the right foot moves forward, look to the right; and when the left foot moves forward, look to the left. Note that the straight line seems to sway in the direction opposite to the movement of the eyes and foot, *i.e.*, when the eyes and foot move to the right, the line seems to move to the left. When the eyes and foot move to the left, the line seems to move to the right. Note that this is done easily, without any hesitation or discomfort.

When you walk, you can imagine that you are looking at the right foot as you step forward with that foot. When you step forward with the left foot, you can imagine that you are looking at your left foot. This can be done in a slow walk or quite rapidly while running straight ahead or in a circle.

DEEP BREATHING

Deep breathing is very effective in improving the accuracy and sensitiveness of the eyes, nerves and mind. The

following suggestions will prove helpful in the practice of
deep breathing: —

1. Avoid all the tight clothing.
2. Open all the windows of the room or select an open
   space free from draught.
3. During breathing keep the mouth closed.
4. Pay more attention to exhalation than inhalation.
5. Avoid quick and jerky breathing.
6. The abdomen should be kept compressed during
   breathing.
7. One must not be satisfied with the few minutes of
   breathing exercises, but one should make a habit of
   conscious deep inspirations and expirations at several
   other times of the day.

BREATHING EXERCISES

VACUUM BREATHING:—Sit comfortably and keep the body
erect. Take in a normal deep breath. When the inhalation
is complete, exhale slowly and with ease. Throw the breath
out in one long, continuous and forceful rhythm. Keep on
exhaling till the last volume of air is out. When this is
done, draw the abdomen in toward the spine and stop
breathing for about five seconds. Then slowly begin to inhale until you get to the normal rhythm of the breath.

ALTERNATE BREATHING: — Sit in an easy posture. Close
the right nostril with the thumb and then slowly inhale
through the left nostril, repeat the word 'Om' four times.

Then firmly close both nostrils by placing forefinger on
the left one and hold the breath in, mentally repeating the
'Om' eight times.

Then remove the thumb from the right nostril, exhale
slowly through that, repeating the 'Om' four times.

As you close the exhalation, draw in the abdomen for-
cibly to expel all the air from the lungs. Then slowly inhale through the right nostril, keeping the left one closed

and after retaining the air, exhale through the left nostril, just as before while repeating 'Om'. Repeat about four times.

The following breathing exercises are quite simple and are performed while standing:—

1. With hands at sides, inhale and exhale slowly and deeply.
2. Stand erect, arms at sides. Inhale, raising the arms forward and upward until the palms touch above the head, at the same time raising on the toes as high as possible. Exhale, lowering the toes, bringing the hands downward in a wide circle until palms touch the thighs.
3. Stand erect, hands at shoulders. Inhale, raising elbows sideways; exhale, bringing elbows down.

CHAPTER XIV

ERRORS OF REFRACTION
MYOPIA

DEFINITION: Myopia has been called near-sightedness, be-cause, in this case, the vision is usually very good for ob-jects which are seen at a near point, while very dim or blurred for objects at ten feet or farther. The eyes are habitually focussed for a point about twelve inches or less. In high degrees of myopia, the eyes may be focussed at less than twelve inches, ten, six, three inches or nearer to the eyes. Some patients can read fine print when held two or three inches. In myopia, the eyeball is elongated.

ACUTE MYOPIA: When myopia is acquired, it is called acute myopia in the early stages. When treated at this time, it is readily curable without glasses. The practice of pres-cribing glasses in these cases leads to a permanent use of them.

PROGRESSIVE MYOPIA: In these cases, the myopia increa-ses quite rapidly, and may be accompanied by much dis-comfort, pain, fatigue and loss of vision. In advanced cases, many become unable to see even with very strong glasses, and can even see better without glasses.

COMPLICATED MYOPIA: Myopia may be complicated with cataract or other eye diseases.

Myopia usually occurs at about twelve years of age. It is rarely congenital. Some become myopic at the age of four, fifteen, seventy or any age, earlier or later. Some children with normal vision may go through life without even be-coming myopic.

It is a popular belief that a habitual use of the eyes for reading, sewing, or for any other use at a near point pro-motes the increase of myopia and that individuals who use their eyes repeatedly for distant vision suffer less from myopia.

But simultaneous retinoscopy always demonstrates that near use of the eyes — even under a strain in a poor light — instead of producing myopia, always lessens it or corrects it altogether; and that a strain to see at a distance always produces myopia.

It can be shown (1) that a strain to see at a distance produces near-sightedness. Look at a Snellen Test Card at twenty feet and read it as well as you can. Now strain or make an effort to see it better, and note that the sight, instead of becoming better, becomes actually worse. (2) That a strain to see at a near point does not increase near-sightedness, but always lessens it. Look at a card of the fine print at six inches from your eyes and read it as well as you can. Now make an effort to see it better, and note that your vision for the near point is lowered, while the ability to read the fine print at a great distance is improved.

CAUSE

PRINCIPAL CAUSE: The principal cause of myopia is staring or making an effort to see at distant objects.

CONTRIBUTING CAUSES: Teachers, parents or others, who use glasses, are under a strain. This strain is contagious, and the children under their care are more apt to acquire myopia than those who are under the care of teachers with normal eyes and normal sight. Constant use of glasses increases myopia. Common sense tells us that as the sight of a myopic patient is good at the near point, the use of glasses will naturally increase the strain.

TREATMENT: Keep in your mind a few facts and practise as instructed in the preceding chapters.

1. All patients who desire to be cured of imperfect sight should discard their glasses and never put them on again for any emergencies. It may be remembered that persons suffering from high myopia are rarely curable but can improve the vision considerably; in such cases glasses may be

used when necessary.

2. Some cases are benefited after other methods have failed by showing the patients how to make their sight worse by staring, straining or making an effort to see. When the cause of the imperfect sight of myopia becomes known, the vision often improves to a considerable degree. When myopic patients learn by actual demonstration the cause of their trouble, it becomes possible for them to improve their sight.

3. Rest of the eyes and mind is the cure for myopia. Any effort to improve the vision always fails. Quite frequently it is difficult for people with imperfect sight to believe that perfect sight requires no effort and that any effort to improve the sight is wrong. It causes habitual strain and it becomes difficult to improve such patients within a short period.

4. Learn first blinking and keeping the lids lowered. If you can make these two fundamentals perfect, then it would be easy for you to improve the eyesight.

5. Practising with a familiar Snellen Test Card is one of the quickest methods of curing myopia temporarily or permanently. The more perfectly the letters of the Snellen Test Card are remembered or imagined, the more completely is the myopia relieved.

6. Children under twelve years of age who have never worn glasses are usually temporarily cured by alternately reading the Snellen Test Card and resting their eyes by palming.

7. Encourage all myopic patients to read the finest print by blinking and keeping the sight on the white spaces. It is a mistake to stop their near work. Badminton and ping-pong are good and useful games for myopic patients.

8. Some persons with imperfect sight have a good imagination, but still their sight is imperfect. Such persons with imperfect sight who have a good imagination fail to use it perfectly all the time; they suppress it and imagine things

imperfectly by an effort which, of course, lowers their vision.

9. Myopia requires a regular and faithful practice. Even when the sight comes to a normal condition, one should continue the practice for some time longer to prevent a relapse. Then one should read the chart daily and stop practice. This will keep him aware about his sight. Whenever there will be any relapse, the patient will correct it himself.

10. Imagination and memory exercises prove most helpful; but when the imagination is poor, swinging and central fixation exercises are a great help. Frequent palming relieves the strain.

11. Reading some small print in dim light for half an hour or so proves very helpful.

CASE REPORTS

THE FOLLOWING CASE REPORTS ARE ONLY SPECIMENS OF MANY MORE THAT ARE EQUALLY INTERESTING.

1. Swami Arjun Deva aged about thirty years, had arrived at the Clinic from Haridwar. The patient could not say whether he was actually born short-sighted; it was discovered at the age of five when he found his distant vision defective. Time passed on without any treatment. At the age of fifteen he was taken to an eye specialist at Nagpur and he was advised to use glasses of -5.0.

The patient continued to pay periodical visits to the best available eye specialists and every two or three years, he had to have his spectacles changed for a stronger pair, until at the age of twenty, he was prescribed glasses of -16.0 for both eyes.

The doctors were of opinion that he should discard his studies and, eventually, he left studies altogether after passing the matriculation.

At the age of twenty-two he left his home in search of some cure for his eyes, and wandered about from place to place. His general health was affected by diabetes. His sight was getting worse and worse. The flying flies appeared before the eyes and this trouble was very annoying to him. Somebody suggested to him to gaze at the sun with open eyes. This increased the discomfort and a new trouble arose. Whenever he stared at an object, the object became distorted and tripled. In the room, everything seemed to be covered with a veil. When he stared at a lamp or a candle, the black and white streaks began to spread on all sides. During this time, he paid visits to an eye specialist of Lahore, and the doctor made it clear to him that the sight was getting worse and prescribed the glasses of -20.0 at the age of thirty. But the glasses neither relieved the troubles nor improved the vision sufficiently.

His sight was rapidly failing. It was a difficulty to read or write anything, despite the enormously powerful glasses he was wearing. He had pains in the head at the slightest attempt to look at anything clearly. No hope of improvement came from any side. Days like a long endless night began to pass. The patient had no further hopes and resigned himself to his fate and waited for death to visit as soon as possible.

One day, the patient happened to see my article on "Throw away your glasses" in the "Hindustan Times." The article encouraged him and gave a ray of hope of recovery.

His vision in the both eyes was 5/200 without glasses and 20/200 with glasses.

With each eye separately, he could not read any letter because soon the letters became double and adopted such a form that he could not distinguish them.

TREATMENT: The first thing I advised the patient was to keep his eyes closed for the most of the time. Next the position of the upper eyelids should always remain lowered; while seeing in front or upward, the lids should not be raised, but the chin, i.e., the position of the upper eyelids should be all the time approximated to that at the time of reading. Now, I demonstrated its efficacy on the chart. When the patient looked at the chart while raising the upper eyelids, the letters became dim, but when he raised the chin, and lowered the upper eyelids, the letters became clearer. Everybody can demonstrate this fact. Keeping the upper eyelids raised is generally seen in myopes and, unless this defect is corrected, it is very difficult to give any benefit to the patient. Lowering the upper eyelids gives rest to the eyes, while raising the upper eyelids causes strain.

The next thing and a very important one was blinking.

For a week, I advised the patient to practise these two fundamental secrets of the cure. After three days, his neck muscles began to ache due to raising the chin all the time. In a week's time, the patient formed a permanent habit, and this was really the secret of his cure. Patients, who cannot obtain this habit of right blinking and lowering the upper eyelids are not benefited permanently.

The trouble of polyopia disappeared and the flying spots appeared only when the patient looked towards a bright light or when he unconsciously stopped blinking.

Second week: I find that myopic patients improve their sight and are cured more quickly by standing near a window and looking off in the distance at large signs or the background behind them. The patient stands with the feet about 12 inches apart before the window and turns the body to the right — at the same time lifting the heel of the left foot. The head and the eyes move with the body. The left heel is then placed on the floor; the body is turned to the left as the patient raises the heel of the right foot. I usually advise the patients to do this right and left swing for a sufficient time. In this swing the nearer objects appear to be moving in the opposite direction, while the farther objects move in the same direction. Some people have a difficulty in practising the swing successfully. They cannot imagine the stationary objects to be moving, no matter how much the swing is practised. They feel absolutely certain that the

stationary object is always stationary and cannot be expected
to move when the body sways from side to side in a long or
short movement. My patient became able to imagine the
objects moving from the very beginning and this helped him
much in improving the sight.

At the end of the second week, I tested the sight and
the vision improved to 10/120, but soon the letters became
double. At once I asked him to close the eyes and to the
right of him I placed the test card on the wall. I called the
patient to come to ten feet distance from the card. I directed
him to blink as he moved his body to the right and to flash
the letter on the test card that he could see without making
an effort of any kind. I explained that the letters could be
seen best by looking a little above or below it, or a little to
the left or right of it. He said that he could see the letters
more clearly when he followed my suggestion, and that the
letters almost disappeared, or became double when he looked
directly at the letter. This method taught him how to see
the objects.

Now from the third week: I gave him sun treatment along
with swinging. Both morning and evening, he faced the sun
with closed eyelids and then moved the body from side to
side, for thirty minutes each time. Just after sun treatment,
he washed the eyes with the lotion "Ophthalmo" and then
began practising swinging. The sun proved to be a miracle
in his case. Daily the vision showed improvement and at the
end of the third week, the vision was 20/40 without glasses.

Now, the patient had no difficulty in going about, and
seeing distant objects. He had grown anxious to improve the
reading sight at an early date. Swamiji was a good writer.
Seeing his interest in this direction, I directed the methods
to improve the near sight. For the distant sight, he continued
the same practices till he left the hospital.

To improve the near sight, I gave him the fundamental
reading card and asked him to hold it at nine inches and
then move the head 1/4 inch from side to side while looking

at the white spaces in between the lines of print, and at the same time to imagine the white lines in between the lines of print to be moving in the opposite direction. Blinking should be at least twice on each line. He could easily do it and then he practised on the books. Then, after three days, I asked him to read the letters and words by blinking on each word. To improve more, he took the help of the sun and now he could read the fine print.

Writing was also difficult task for him. I asked him to draw only lines like ΛΛ moving the sight up and down with the point of the pen, blinking on each line. After a few days' practice, he could read and write very well.

2. His Excellency The Senior Commanding General of Nepal began to use glasses of -5.0 from the age of 8 years, and paid periodical visits to best available eye specialists in India and England, and every now and then he had to have his spectacles changed for a stronger pair until at the age of 48 he was prescribed glasses of -8.0. The last doctor had informed him that the vision was very poor even with glasses; and though the number of glasses came to -12.0 yet the vision was the same with -8.0 or with -12.0, hence he thought it better to prescribe the glasses of the lower power. The sight was rapidly failing in spite of the constant use of glasses. No hope of improvement came from any side.

His Excellency came to know about me and my system of treatment through his relative and called me at Nepal. The examination revealed the following facts:

Vision Test	Without glasses.		Without glasses.	
	Distant Vision	Near Vision	Distant Vision	Near Vision
Both eyes	$\frac{20}{200}$	J 3 at 9 inches.	$\frac{20}{70}$	J 1 at 9 inches.
Right eye	$\frac{10}{200}$	J 4 at 9 inches.	$\frac{20}{200}$	J 2 at 9 inches.
Left eye	$\frac{20}{200}$	J 3 at 9 inches.	$\frac{20}{70}$	J 1 at 9 inches.

TREATMENT: First I educated him in blinking and advised to keep the eyes closed all the time as far as possible, and to open the eyes only slightly (half open) in case of a necessity, and to keep the body swinging gently from side to side all the time.

At bed time, a little warm milk-cream was applied on the eyes.

MORNING AND EVENING:

(a) Sun treatment and massage of the forehead with oleum. The patient faced the sun with the eyes closed and moved the body gently from side to side for 15 minutes. At this time, I used to rub a little oleum on the forehead and then massage the forehead in the following way:

FOREHEAD MASSAGE: Place the left hand gently on the head and the right hand fingers (index, middle and ring fingers) on the forehead. Ask the patient to keep the eyes closed and move gently from side to side. The fingers remain in position. The patient feels the fingers to be moving in the opposite direction. At intervals, the patient is asked to keep the imagination on the fingers. After a few minutes only, the patient feels relaxed and begins to doze. All headache and strain are relieved in no time.

The following errors one has to safeguard oneself from in

order to obtain the maximum benefits from this treatment (Forehead massage).

1. Pressure on the head may be much.

2. The patient may not keep the imagination on the fingers but remember some other episodes.

3. There may be some noise or something else which may disturb the patient's mind.

4. The instructor may begin to move the fingers with the movement of the patient.

5. The patient may begin to move with jerks and strain. This massage was given while H. E. took sun treatment.

(b) After finishing sun treatment and massage, the eyes were washed with cold water and 20 drops of Ophthalmo.

(c) After finishing the eye bath, H. E. practised *Touch Swing* and swinging exercises before the bars and chart. Right methods of reading and writing were given.

On the last day of treatment the followng directions were laid down for His Excellency:

DIRECTIONS: 1. Use of glasses only to see distant objects when necessity arises.

2. Dark glasses should not be used. If it is too bright, then Crooks A may be used.

3. Near work should be done without glasses at the convenient distance.

4. Remember three points to avoid the strain:

a. Upper lids should be kept lowered.

b. Gentle blinking all the time.

c. Imagine stationary objects moving in the opposite direction while walking or riding.

5. Whenever there is heaviness in the forehead or eyes, close the eyes and practise touch swing for a few minutes.

6. Sun treatment, eye-wash and touch swing should be practised daily morning and evening.

7. Write the conditon of the eyes to the doctor every fortnight.

Now, the record of vision was again taken:

Without Glasses

	D. V.	N. V.
B. E.	$\dfrac{20}{100}$	J 2 at 9 inches
R. E.	$\dfrac{20}{200}$	J 3 at 9 inches
L. E.	$\dfrac{20}{100}$	J 2 at 9 inches

With Glasses

	D. V.	N. V.
B. E.	$\dfrac{20}{30}$	J 1 at 9 inches
R. E.	$\dfrac{20}{70}$	J 1 at 9 inches
L. E.	$\dfrac{20}{30}$	J 1 at 9 inches

Now, the vision was much better. The eyes could open very well and could easily stand for the bright lights. There was no difficulty in the daily routine without glasses. The expression of the face looked brighter. Others also could note that the eyes looked much better. His Highness The Maharaja of Nepal had remarked: "Your eyes seem to have much improved."

After six months, I was again called to give another course of treatment, for one month. In the morning, I put him on sun treatment, forehead massage, eye-wash, palming and swinging exercise No. 5 and central fixation. Gradually the vision of each eye went on improving and the results were: —

Without Glasses

| R. E. | $\dfrac{20}{40}$ | J 1 at 9 inches |
| L. E. | $\dfrac{20}{30}$ | J 1 at 9 inches |

With Glasses

| R. E. | $\dfrac{20}{20}$ | J 1 at 12 inches |
| L. E. | $\dfrac{20}{20}$ | J 1 at 12 inches |

After two years, His Excellency wrote that his vision was so good that he could shoot at a long distance without glasses. His Excellency wrote in his remark:

"I was using glasses of -8.0.... It is simply marvellous that, within a short time, the visual power of my eyes has wonderfully increased...."

"My daughter, who was using glasses of -3.0 cylindrical, was able to discard the glasses and to gain normal vision after 6 days' treatment."

"This time, the vision improved still further. From 20ft. distance, I have been able to read 30ft. line without glasses, and 20ft. line with glasses. The right eye had very poor chances of its improvement, but it has now improved to the level of the left eye. My relative had blindness in his right eye, and was all right in a week's time.

"In the interest of suffering humanity, I feel it is my duty to give expression to my deep sense of gratitude to Dr. Agarwal...."

3. A male patient aged 18 of -3.5 was able to read the top letter of pocket eye testing chart without glasses, that is, his vision was 10/50. First I demonstrated how to blink, then gave sun treatment for 15 minutes and asked him to practise palming for 10 minutes. While palming, he could imagine perfectly. When he opened his eyes, he began to read the next lines of the chart. When he began to read the third line of the chart, he began to stare, so I asked him to close his eyes and palm again. After 5 minute's, palming, he began to read the chart again. I asked him to close the eyes for a second after reading each letter and palm for 2 minutes after reading each line. This checked his staring. In half an hour's practice, he was able to read five feet line from five feet, vision became 5/5, that is, normal.

This improvement gave him great encouragement and he continued the practices for several months but was unable to make the improvement permanent. The reason was that he could not keep the upper eyelids in the right position and could not blink frequently at other times. He could relax perfectly only at the time of practice. Then he wanted to give up the practices and use glasses. So I advised him to use -3.0 glass for the distance only, and practise sun treatment and palming every morning to check further deterioration.

4. A male patient, aged 23 began to use glasses of -1.5 from the age of 13, and the number gradually went on increasing to -7.0, in spite of constant use of specs. He stayed in the clinic for 10 days as an indoor patient. From the first day, he kept the lids down, did not try to look up or in front, and blinked frequently just in the normal way. One day, his friend came to see him. While talking, he looked at the ground and not at his friend. He explained to his friend that this position of upper eyelids checks strain, helps in the improvement of vision and I should follow my doctor. The patient wrote "Blink",

"Blink" on several pieces of cardboards and put them on the table, walls and on his coat. This helped him to blink all the time.

With closed eyes, his imagination was poor, so I put him on swinging exercises. Glasses were discarded permanently. Vision began to improve and he was able to read fifty feet line 5, C, G, O at 10 ft. distance and the vision was 10/50. After 2 years, he wrote, "I had been quite regular in my practices. Recently, I got my eyes tested by the local doctor, who prescribed glasses of -2.5. As I am still unable to see distinctly at the black-board in the college, I want to use glasses for distance only, but I would not give up my practices."

5. A college student, using glasses of -5.5, wanted treatment. I used to attend on him at his residence. I advised him not to use glasses at all. His vision was 10/200 without glasses and 10/30 with glasses. By sun treatment, palming and swinging, he was able to read 10/30 on the very first day and felt his head and eyes very light. In the noon, he went to the college for about an hour and could not check the temptation of using glasses. When he returned home, he got severe headache. Next day, when he described his story, I said that it was a great mistake and it would be difficult now to improve due to the severe reaction. After five days' trial, the patient did not show any good improvement and the case was given up.

6. A girl had myopic astigmatism and was using glasses of -3.0 cylindrical. She was able to imagine a black dot at varying distances. Game of ball was a great help. Sun treatment relieved the glare. After six days' treatment, she gained normal vision and discarded the glasses permanently. At times, specially in dim light, she felt her distant sight defective, but she overcame this defect by the imagination of "O".

GAME OF BALL: Sit by the side of a table. Cover the eyes with the left hand. Roll a wooden ball on the table to the opposite side. Someone helps from the opposite side. Concentrate the mind on the sound which is produced when the ball rolls. Catch the ball when it comes to your side, by hearing its sound. After playing for a few minutes remove the left hand, read the chart while still playing with the ball. Repeat several times.

7. A school teacher was using glasses of -2.5 and was very anxious to discard them. His thoughts were distorted and it was impossible for him to practise with concentration. While palming or swinging, he had such thoughts as one generally has in dreams. I changed his exercises every now and then and he tried the treatment for one month regularly, but did not show any improvement. Improvement in such cases is generally not possible due to a lack of good imagination.

8. Amna, a lovely girl of 10 used to stare and complained to her mother that she could not see the letters on the blackboard in the class-room clearly. She had myopia and was able to read the thirty feet line at 10 ft. distance. When she read the chart, she did not blink even once and bent her head forward.

First, I taught her blinking and instructed her mother to put her under sun treatment, palming and chart reading. After one week, her mother brought her for an eye examination, but Amna did not show any improvement. I said to Amna, "If you learn to blink all the time, your eyesight will be all right within a week." Her mother said, "Amna, you will get a prize if you can learn blinking." Amna promised to learn blinking. This time, I advised Amna to practise swinging before bars for 10 minutes four times a day. This exercise was like a game to her and she liked it much. Amna did not come on the seventh day, as her mother was very busy in other affairs. Then, I called Amna on the telephone and enquired how she was. She replied, "I am all right now and can read 10ft. line at 20ft. distance". I said, "How did you improve so much with-

in a few days?" She replied, "Because now I blink." Since
then, Amna blinks all the time and educates other children
to blink. Her mother was very grateful for the benefit.

9. One student was wearing glasses of -4.0 and the vision was 10/100. He was ready to discard the glasses permanently and practise faithfully. He could read finest print
at six inches, but central fixation was poor, that is,
he could not see each letter or word regarded blacker than
the rest. First, I put him on central fixation series and improved his central fixation at six inches, because at this distance, his vision was best. Then I placed a Snellen Test
Card at 1 foot to practise central fixation and gradually increased its distance to 10 feet according to the progress in
central fixation. Occasionally, he practised palming and
swinging. On the tenth day, his vision was 10/30. Then
he went away home and informed me after three months
that he could read then 20ft. line at 20 feet distance.

10. A student had myopia of about -3.0 in the right
eye and -3.5 in the left eye with a little cylinder. The vision was 20/200 in each eye. By sun treatment and palming, he improved his sight to 20/70.

Then, I put the chart at three feet and asked him to
practise central fixation. When he looked at the top of C,
he noted the bottom of C worse, and *vice-versa*. By frequent palming, he could practise central fixation on the
seventh line (2, Q, C, O, G, D, C). Next step was to imagine
a black dot in the bottom part of each letter. When he
was able to imagine the dot, the letter became blacker and
began to pulsate up and down or from side to side. Gradually, the distance of the chart was increased to ten feet
and the sight improved to 10/20. Beyond this, he began
to strain. I changed the practice and asked him to read the
photo print at six inches and the big chart at 12 feet alternately, or to look at the tip of the finger at six inches
and the chart at 12 feet alternately.

During palming, he could not get a good relaxation, so I

suggested to him, "Imagine a black screen, and place a white handkerchief on this black screen. Place the letter T in the centre of the handkerchief and imagine as if the letter T does drill. When it stretches the arms up, it becomes Y, and then again assumes its position of T. When it brings the right arm down and stretches it to the left, it becomes F. He could perfectly imagine like this, and the vision improved to 10/15 or 20/30.

11. A young man was using glasses of -2.0 Spherical and the vision of each eye was 20/100 or 6/36 in meters approximately. He appeared in the competitive examination of the railways, in which the standard of vision required without glasses was 6/9 in one eye and 6/12 in the other eye. He had a brilliant career but the defective vision was a great obstacle in his way. He asked me for help in choosing the best method of treatment to improve his eyesight.

Rest of the eyes and mind was the cure for myopia. Any effort to see or to improve the vision always fails. How were people with myopia conscious of a strain? This was a very important question. When methods were practised in the wrong way or practised unsuccessfully, a strain or effort to see better could usually be felt or demonstrated.

Quite frequently it is difficult for people with imperfect sight to believe that perfect sight requires no effort and that any effort to improve the sight is wrong. They forget that the normal function of the eyes is, like the function of other sensory organs, without effort.

I directed the young man to sit with the eyes closed and covered with the palms of each hand in such a way as to avoid pressure on the eyeball. At the end of half an hour, he was directed to stand with the feet about one foot apart and sway from side to side, paying no attention to the apparent movement of stationary objects. He moved his body, head and eyes to the same direction and regulated his movements with his breathing. When he swayed to the right he inhaled; and when he swayed to the left he exhaled.

Practice of palming and swinging produced a sense of
relaxation in his eyes and mind. The next procedure was
to improve his memory and imagination which if practised
correctly is a great help for the improvement of vision. The
patient while blinking gently for a few seconds, looked at
one letter of the Snellen Test Card which had been committed to memory. The letter looked at appeared best.
When he closed his eyes, he remembered a known letter
and the picture of the letter was quite vivid in his imagination. Observing that his imagination was good I expected
that he would show a considerable and permanent improvement in his eyesight. I have frequently observed that persons with a high degree of near-sightedness do not improve
much until the memory or imagination of one known letter
has improved to a considerable degree. It is interesting to
demonstrate in these cases that the more perfectly a letter
is remembered or imagined, the better becomes the sight.
When a letter is remembered or imagined as well with the
eyes opened as with the eyes closed, a maximum amount
of improvement in the vision is obtained.

The smaller a letter remembered or imagined the better the vision. A full stop or a tiny dot is usually preferable but I advised this patient to remember a colon (:).
While the eyes are closed or open, the top dot should be
imagined best while the lower dot is more or less blurred
and not seen so well. In a few moments it is well to shift
and imagine the lower dot best while the upper dot is imagined not so well. Common sense makes it evident that
one dot cannot be imagined best unless there is some other
dot or other object which is seen worse.

The patient remembered the colon perfectly, shifting constantly from one dot to the other. Sometimes he prefered
to remember a semicolon. He thought that the memory of
a very small colon would be more difficult than the memory
of a large one, but he soon realized that the very small
colon was remembered best.

He kept the chart at 5 feet and recalled the memory of
the colon and shifted his sight from one small letter to the
other without making an effort to see. Each letter appeared
very black and distinct. Then he gradually increased the
distance to twenty feet and shifted his sight on the twenty
feet line while keeping the memory of the colon.

The improvement on the twenty feet line was temporary,
that is, he could see this line at twenty feet distance only when
he could remember the colon or a dot well. However, his
improvement was remarkable. He could read 6/9 and 6/12
quite easily, and he was very glad when he passed the
medical test of the Railway Board.

CHAPTER XV

ERRORS OF REFRACTION

HYPERMETROPIA

Hypermetropia or far sight is supposed to be congenital; but the truth is that this condition is acquired by the strain to see at the near point. It is sometimes acquired soon after birth, or it may manifest at ten, twenty, thirty, or forty years of age. Eighty percent of eye troubles are caused by hypermetropia, while nearsightedness occurs in ten per cent. There are only ten per cent of normal eyes. These figures are startling. The majority of persons at the age of forty or over acquire hypermetropia.

In hypermetropia the sight at the near point is usually poor. When the distant sight is good for distant vision, that does not necessarily mean that the sight is also good for reading at a near point of ten or twelve inches. Too often such cases are not treated seriously. Poor sight for reading is usually corrected by the use of reading glasses.

In middle age, serious eye diseases are caused by hypermetropia. Among the most common are glaucoma, cataract and diseases of the optic nerve and retina. In the early stages of these serious diseases, they are more rapidly curable than after they become chronic and more serious, because the vision is only slightly affected and the treatment which cures the hypermetropia is the treatment which prevents serious eye diseases. It should be emphasized that an early treatment of hypermetropia yields quicker, and more permanent results than later treatment.

The best methods of preventing hypermetropia are palming and reading fine print, and imagining stationary objects to be moving. Imagination of white spaces in between the lines of print is a very useful method for the cure of hypermetropia.

All measures which prevent strain and promote relaxation, are always beneficial. A strain at a near point always increases the amount of hypermetropia or produces it in the normal eye while a strain to see at a distance lessens hypermetropia and the vision may improve and continue to improve until myopia is produced, when the vision is lowered. Some patients stare towards the moon. Out of them, those who are hypermetropic improve; but those who are myopic become more defective. If distant sight is good, central fixation exercises will be sufficient to improve the near sight. If distant sight is also defective, first improve the distant vision by swinging exercises and palming. Blinking on white lines and reading of fine print card with a card hole during the course of treatment prove very helpful. Kite flying, shooting, tennis, running are good exercises. Frequent visits to the movies prove very beneficial. Concentration on candle flame while counting 100 respirations is very helpful.

CASE REPORTS

1. A boy of nine years had difficulty in reading his book. An eye specialist prescribed glasses of plus 6.0 for each eye. The father did not like the idea of putting on spectacles on the face of the young child, so he brought him to me for treatment. I prescribed sun treatment, palming and reading of Snellen Eye Chart and reading test type. The boy practised under the care of his father morning and evening for half an hour. Within a month's time, his eyesight became normal both for the distance and the near.

2. A college student was wearing glasses of plus 5.5 constantly. One of his doctor friends told him that he might suffer from glaucoma in his old age. He came for my opinion. I said, "It may become true. If you would go under my treatment, you would improve your eyesight."

Without glasses, his vision of each eye was 20/70 for the distance, and No.1 on fundamental card for the near point.

He attended the clinic daily for 20 days and repeated the following programme every day:

1. Apply Resolvent 200 with a rod in each eye.
2. Sun treatment for 15 minutes.
3. Eye-wash with cold water.
4. Palming for 5 minutes.
5. Swinging before bars with both eyes for 10 minutes.
6. Central fixation exercises for 20 minutes.
7. Reading of distant chart for 5 minutes.
8. Reading of reading test type and book for 10 minutes, in good light and candle light.

He repeated the same programme at his home.

After twenty days, his vision was —

R. E. 20/30 No. 6 of the fundamentals card.

L. E. 20/30 No. 6 of the fundamentals card.

The patient had to study for some competitive examination and wanted glasses, so glasses of plus 2.5 for reading only were prescribed and he was able to read more easily than with his former glasses. He continued sun treatment, palming and reading of the fundamentals card daily for 20 minutes.

3. A young female patient complained to her doctor that she felt pain in the eyeballs and a heaviness in the head while doing sewing and needle work. The doctor prescribed glasses of plus 0.75 for each eye; but she got no relief. She again went to the doctor who advised her to continue the same glasses for sometime. When she found no benefit, she came to my clinic. The examination revealed that she had normal sight both for the distance and the near point. Then I gave her a needle and thread to sew in my presence. While sewing, she neither blinked nor shifted her sight with the movement of the needle, but stared continuously at the stitches. I demonstrated the right method of sewing. At first, she showed shyness and felt

little difficulty, but then soon she brought it into her habit, and did the sewing for an hour without any discomfort. Since then, she made no complaint about her eyes.

4. Mr. Gupta, a college student used to feel eye strain and headache in reading. Sometimes reading of a page became difficult. He used glasses of plus 0.5 with a little cylinder under the advice of an eye specialist, for several months. He could read 20 feet line at twenty feet distance, and finest print at one foot distance. First, I taught him to blink on the white lines in between the lines of print and he repeated this exercise on 10 pages several times a day. After 3 days I gave him a pocket C card to practise central fixation. On the sixth day, I asked him to keep his sight on the white line just below a word and imagine it blacker, and finish 2 pages in this way. From the seventh day, he began reading his book with a card hole. On the tenth day, he read his book for hours together without any discomfort. He put a question:

"How is it that I got eyestrain while reading though my sight was normal, and how did central fixation help me so much?"

"Your eyes tried to see many a word at a glance and this caused strain. Central fixation taught your eyes to see each word at a time."

5. A male patient used to get severe pain in his right eye for 5 years. The pain usually increased in reading to such an extent that even a few minutes' reading was not possible. The doctors prescribed plus glasses which could not stop the pain. The patient had to discontinue his studies.

His vision was normal both for the distance and the near point. For a few days, I put him on the swinging exercise, which gave him relief and the pain became much less. Then I asked him to practise central fixation on "C" chart, pocket size, and blink on the white lines imagining the letters above the white line blacker. Then I gave a photoprint card to read with both eyes and each eye separately. The patient was totally relieved of the trouble and was able to read for hours without feeling any strain.

The cause of severe pain in the right eye was loss of central fixation while reading. When the eye began to see the letters with central fixation, the strain was relieved.

6. A young man of thirty complained of redness, pain and watering in his eye while reading. He had worn glasses of plus one for several years and for a time they helped him in his work. After some illness, he found that his eyesight was further impaired and the glasses did not relieve the discomforts.

I tested his sight with the test cards and found the vision of each eye 10/20. He stared at every letter that he read. When he was reading, the watery condition increased. His sight was first tested with a white card with black letters and later with a black card with white letters. He read equally well with both cards. He could read the sentence number 3 of the Fundamental card without glasses.

I gave him the sun treatment using my sun glass rapidly on his closed eyelids. After facing the sun for about ten minutes he practised palming and then practised on the Snellen Test Card from 5 to 10 feet. I explained to him some facts to prevent staring.

When the normal eye has normal sight it never tries to see, it is at rest. When it is at rest it is always moving or shifting, it never stares. Shifting may be done consciously with improvement in the vision. To improve imperfect sight by shifting it is well to move the head and eyes from one side of a letter to the other side, while the letter is imagined to be moving in the opposite direction. When the shifting is slow, short, and easy, the best results in the improvement of the vision are obtained. Any attempt to stop the shifting lowers the vision.

The patient practised shifting correctly from side to side of a letter. The letter appeared to move in the opposite direction and appeared more distinct than the other letters not directly regarded. Soon the vision began to improve and in half an hour's treatment he was able to read 10/10. The eyes became light and the redness became less.

To improve the reading sight I gave him the photographic print and directed him to shift his sight from side to side on the white lines in between the lines of print and then read the sentences of the fundamentals card alternately. While practising he blinked gently on every line. It was interesting that he soon began to read the fine print of the Fundamentals card.

The patient continued the practice at his home and after a week it was found that his distant sight was 10/10 and he could now read the photographic print and suffered from no discomfort in the eyes.

7. A lady aged 18 years used to suffer from headache and strain while reading. Her glasses of plus 0.5 always increased the trouble. When I asked her to read she held the book at about 20 inches. I said, "Are you an old lady?"

"Why do you say like that, doctor."

"Because you hold the book at a distance from where old people see best. You will see best at 10 or 12 inches distances," I said.

When she held the book at 12 inches, she could read quite comfortably for long hours, and this little hint cured her permanently. She was advised to read fine print in good light and candle light alternately.

CHAPTER XVI

ERRORS OF REFRACTION

ASTIGMATISM

The study of astigmatism is important because of its frequency and because so many serious eye diseases are preceded by astigmatism. The eye specialists tell their patients that in order to prevent serious eye diseases, glasses should be worn constantly. Such patients, accordingly, become much worried and are in constant fear of serious eye troubles developing, and probable blindness resulting. It is true that the glasses prescribed may give a relief; but usually patients are not benefited very much by the use of glasses.

OCCURRENCE: Astigmatism is one of the most common defects of the human eye. Most people with astigmatism have had it since birth. In some cases, it may increase, while in other cases, it may become less or entirely disappear. Astigmatism is usually combined with hypermetropia or myopia. Some cases of astigmatism are due to imperfect curvature of the lens, or less frequently to a malformation of the eyeball.

SYMPTOMS: When a high degree of astigmatism is present, the vision is appreciably lowered. Usually when vertical lines are regarded, they may appear more distinct than the horizontal lines, or the reverse may be the case. This is, however not a reliable test because patients with a normal vision do not always see vertical or horizontal lines equally well.

Many patients with astigmatism complain of headaches and pain in various parts of the head and eyes. Some patients have said that when their eyes become tired or when they feel uncomfortable in any way, they get relief by removing the glasses. One patient after wearing glasses for a few days, complained that every morning, when he put his glasses on, the pain in his head increased very much, and that, after wearing glasses for a few hours, the pain was partially relieved. His doctor told him that he needed to wear the glasses several weeks before his eyes could get used to them. The patient then told him that he had come to have glasses fitted to his eyes, and not his eyes fitted to glasses.

CAUSE: Astigmatism is caused by mental strain or an effort to see, either consciously or unconsciously. It has been demonstrated that astigmatism can be produced by staring or straining to see. The normal eye with normal sight, normal memory or normal imagination has no astigmatism, but when the normal eye remembers or imagines imperfectly, the retinoscope shows the presence of astigmatism.

Pain in the eyes and the head can always be produced in the normal eye by straining or making an effort to see. Such headaches disappear promptly when relaxation methods are employed.

TREATMENT: Astigmatism is caused by a mental strain and can only be cured by a complete relief of the strain.

Patients suffering from various forms of astigmatism are benefited by practising central fixation, swinging, improving memory, sun treatment and by the art of seeing view-cards.

For the correction of astigmatism, we should consider favourable conditions, which promote the best vision. Some patients with astigmatism, perhaps the majority, prefer bright light. They can see better in the strong sunlight and the astigmatism becomes less when the light is good. Other patients with astigmatism see better, and the astigmatism becomes less or disappears in a dim light, while it may be very much increased in a bright light. Some patients give good results on a black chart while others on a white chart. The patient should practise on the chart on which he gets better results. For the improvement of the near sight, central fixation series are very helpful and for the distant sight swinging generally is very beneficial. Imagination of a black dot is a great help in many cases.

A boy of sixteen was treated by me for the relief of eye troubles, caused by a compound hypermetropic astigmatism. Sunlight caused great discomfort to him and he suffered from headache. He also complained of seeing floating specks. He was not able to read his books for any length of time without pain and fatigue. His distant vision was also imperfect. He went to different eye specialists for the relief of the eye troubles. Each doctor prescribed a different number for his glasses; but no one could help him in relieving the trouble.

I tested his sight without glasses. The vision of the right eye was 10/100 and the vision of the left eye was 10/70. He could not read any print of the reading test type, and as he tried to read wrinkles appeared on his forehead and cheeks.

The first treatment was to give him sun treatment in the early morning for 10 to 30 minutes and then he palmed for 10 minutes continuously. After three days' practice he felt himself better. Then I educated him in blinking for about fifteen minutes. Distant buildings seen through the window appeared to move slightly with him, while the window and its bars moved rapidly opposite. Whenever he stopped blinking to see the things better, the movement of objects became less or stopped altogether and this caused discomfort. I told him to close the eyes at once for a few minutes whenever he felt discomfort. He continued this swaying practice daily for four or five times. Swinging helped him very much in relieving all kinds of his discomforts, the vision also improved both for the distance and the near. Seven days later his vision as noted by the test card had improved to 10/20 and the letters were clearer and more distinct. I gave him a reading test type to hold in his hand. He could read No. 5 of the fundamentals easily.

Along with the sway, he practised sun treatment and palming daily. Just after palming he practised on the reading test type. After a fortnight he became able to read the fine print. Daily he was advised to write the whole reading test type five times.

2. A girl of eighteen came to me for treatment. She began to use glasses from the age of seven for slight convergent squint in the left eye. At the age of fifteen no squint was appreciable, but she could produce it by effort. Her doctor changed the glasses and prescribed a lower number. Since then she was using this number. She was using glasses of simple myopic astigmatism.

I examined her thoroughly in the dark room and on the test card; and found that she was suffering from simple hypermetropic astigmatism and not with simple myopic astigmatism. Her vision on the test card was 10/5 and she could read only No. 5 of the reading test type. She felt pain and headache whenever she read even if it be for a short time.

I demonstrated blinking to her for some minutes and then asked her to glance at the white spaces in between the words for two days. During these two days she finished about 100 pages, glancing at white spaces and felt no trouble. Then on the third day I gave her the test type, and she read the whole of it. It was very pleasing to her. Then I gave the reduced photographic type; she felt her eyes tired. I asked her to palm for 10 minutes and the eyes became very restful.

3. Another girl aged twelve, daughter of a civil surgeon, was suffering from compound myopic astigmatism. She was using glasses for five years. Her vision was 10/100 with each eye separately and with both eyes together. In every case blinking and lowering the upper eyelids are the first

instructions to be given. I asked her to practise the sway before the window for four days continuously four times a day each time devoting half an hour. She practised the sway very well both with closed and open eyes. On the fifth day I examined her again on the test card; her vision was 10/40 this day.

Then I advised her to take the sun treatment, before practising the sway. The sun helped her very much. By the twelfth day her vision improved to 10/15.

4. A student aged seventeen wanted to be treated for mixed astigmatism by correspondence. He had studied my literature very well. I agreed to give him the treatment by correspondence, because he was a boy and could not come from Deccan to my office. He had great faith in my treatment. The glasses that he was using gave him pain. With the aid of palming, swinging, and the use of his imagination, his vision improved to normal. Each letter contained many pages, full of questions. It is very unusual for such patients to obtain such quick cure by correspondence.

5. A patient, a European girl of seventeen complained of feeling of dust and glare in the sun, dimness before the eyes when she came from the light into the shade, sight defective both for the distance and the near point, frequent headache and heaviness in the eyes. An eye specialist had prescribed the following glasses:

Right eye: plus 0.75 Spherical with plus 0.5 Cylindrical,
Left eye: plus 2.5 Spherical with plus 0.5 Cylindrical.

After using these glasses for six months she threw them away as they did not relieve her complaints and disfigured the face.

On the advice of a friend, she attended my clinic with her father. The examination revealed the following facts:

1. Distant Vision of the right eye=10/40
    Distant Vision of the left eye=10/200
    Near Vision of the right eye at 9 inches=No. 7 of
                            the Fundamentals Card.

Near Vision of the left eye at 9 inches=No. 2 of
the Fundamentals Card.

2. No improvement with glasses.
3. Field of vision much contracted in both eyes.
4. Deficiency of Vitamin A, as indicated by Bio-Photo-
meter.
5. No organic defect.

I prescribed the following treatment which she daily
carried out at home and in the clinic:

1. Sun treatment with eye-wash.
2. Palming for 5 minutes.
3. Swinging exercises.
4. Reading the Chart at 10 feet and reading test type
at 9 inches in good light and in candle light.
5. At times central fixation exercises and game of snap.

After 20 days' treatment the right eye became normal,
and the left improved to 10/40. She was able to read No.
7 of fundamental card with the left eye. Field of vision
became normal in each eye. All other complaints disappeared.

The attention was concentrated now on the left eye. I
advised her to cover the good eye with an eye-shield for
most of the time, and continue the exercises with the left
eye. The improvement was steady, and after two months'
treatment, left eye also became normal. She used to read
photo-print with each eye.

6. A student was suffering from mixed astigmatism, that
is, in each eye the number of glasses was plus and minus.
His vision from twenty feet was 20/50 without glasses, and
20/30 with glasses. He felt great strain in reading and frequently suffered from headache and often saw floating specks
appearing before his eyes.

In astigmatism the eyeball adopts an irregular curvature.
Like other errors of refraction astigmatism is also acquired
and it frequently changes its axis and its number. To believe that astigmatism is permanent and congenital is wrong.

This patient had several prescriptions of glasses and each differed from the other.

Like myopia and hypermetropia astigmatism is caused by an effort to see. The greater the strain, the more imperfect becomes the vision. The patient had the habit of looking at objects by lowering the chin and raising the eyeballs. In reading also he had adopted the staring habit. Every one who looked at his eyes said that his way of looking at objects was very unusual. Blinking was absent. The harder he tried to look at objects, the greater the discomfort he felt in his eyes.

Rest when properly employed cures all forms of imperfect sight. The great difficulty is that all people are not able to rest their eyes properly. It has been found that the tendency of most people is to concentrate or strain. When one letter of the Snellen Test Card is regarded continuously, imperfect sight is produced. Trying to keep the eye immovable causes imperfect sight.

I demonstrated to him how the normal eye looked at objects without effort and shifted itself rapidly and blinked frequently; but it was difficult for him to adopt the right habit, hence there was no improvement for one week. One of the successful methods for myopic and astigmatic cases is, "Make the sight worse by a strong effort to stare or by trying to see the top and bottom parts of the big 'C' equally well at a time." The patient increased his effort to stare consciously and felt manifest strain in his head and all his nerves and realized the harm it could produce.

To such patients the long swing is a very good method to begin with. By practising the long swing properly, fatigue is relieved as well as pain, headache and other discomforts. The sway always brings about a relief from the effort of trying to see, staring or concentration. But good things which are done by the patient do not always succeed. He stood with feet nine inches apart. When he swayed to the right, the whole weight was on the right leg and the heel of the left foot was raised; and when he swayed to the left, the whole weight of the body was on the left leg and the right heel was raised. While practising the sway he moved his eyes in one direction and his head in the opposite direction, the result was a very bad strain which was very painful. The right thing was to move the eyes and head in the same direction along with the movement of the body. When he practised the sway properly, his pain disappeared. A Snellen Test Card was then placed in front of him at five feet distance. When he moved his head and eyes a short distance from side to side, the test card appeared to move in the opposite direction.

The long swing enabled him to practise the short swing. When he moved his head and eyes slowly, gently and properly from side to side of or above and below each letter without an effort to see the letter, the letter appeared to move in the opposite direction. He also observed that the letter which appeared to move in the opposite direction was more distinct than the other letters. But whenever he stared at the letter while shifting his sight from side to side or above and below it, the letter appeared stationary and central fixation was lost.

The memory of familiar objects with the eyes closed is a great help in obtaining a relaxation to the eyes and lessening the amount of astigmatism. Perfect memory of an object means perfect sight, because the greater the relaxation the quicker does the astigmatism disappear. It often happens that patients with astigmatism find it difficult to obtain a relaxation, because they try to see or imagine too much of any one object at once. To this patient, palming or the memory of familiar objects did not help as he always made an effort to bring a perfect picture of an object.

Short sway while sitting on a chair gave him a feeling of good relaxation. When he swayed a little to the right he felt as if his legs placed on the ground appeared to move to the left and *vice versa*. So instead of palming he preferred the short sway with closed eyes. At times he placed his finger opposite the lower part of the chin and then moved his head and eyes from side to side. When he did the short sway properly, he could imagine the finger to be moving.

He practised various central fixation exercises as given in the book quite successfully, but when I asked him to read the fine print card, he hesitated to read it. He believed that fine print reading may cause strain and myopia. I told him that the Chinese used a very large print and suffered most from myopia. Large print instead of being a rest to the eyes was a great strain. Fine print could not be read clearly or easily when an effort was made. When the eyes looked directly at the letters, an effort was required, while looking at the white spaces between the lines was a rest, and by practice in this way, one could become able to see the letters clearly, without looking directly at them. When he looked at the white spaces between the lines of print or ordinary book type, he could read for hours and no fatigue, pain or discomfort was felt.

After a month's treatment he could read the 20 feet line easily without glasses. He could read the photoprint without any difficulty. The expression of his eyes was completely changed. The upper eyelids were kept lowered. The eyes gave a calm and quiet expression. The muscles of the face seemed to be relaxed indicating no wrinkles.

Reading of fine print in candle light proved extremely beneficial.

CHAPTER XVII

PRESBYOPIA OR OLD AGE SIGHT

When most people with normal eyes arrive at the age of forty and upwards, they usually have difficulty in reading books or newspapers, although their sight for distance may be normal; and they are dependent upon their glasses for reading. This condition has been called old age sight, although it could be defined more accurately as the imperfect sight of middle age. The medical term for this form of imperfect sight is presbyopia.

The decline of near vision with advancing years is thought to be the normal result of growing old. The cause is said to be due to the hardening of the lens of the eye to such an extent that focus of the eye cannot be brought to a near point on account of the inability of the hard lens to change its shape.

The eye is one of the sense organs, and when other sense organs do not grow old, then, why should the eye lose its sight with advancing years? Many persons at forty can read fine print at four inches without glasses, and they show normal sight on the distant chart also. There are people who refuse to become presbyopic at all. There are also people who regain their near vision after having lost it for ten, fifteen, or more years; and there are people who, while presbyopic for some objects, have a perfect sight for others. Many dressmakers, for instance, can thread a needle with the naked eye, and yet they cannot read or write without glasses.

The truth about presbyopia is that it is not "a normal result of growing old", being both preventable and curable. It is not caused by hardening of the lens, but by a strain to see at the near point. It has no necessary connection with age, since it occurs, in some cases, as early as ten years, while in others it never occurs at all. It is true that the lens does harden with advancing years; but since the lens is not a factor in accommodation, this fact is immaterial. Presbyopia is, in fact, simply a form of hypermetropia in which the vision for the near point is chiefly affected. When a person with presbyopia tries to read the fine print and fails, the focus is always pushed farther away than it was before the attempt was made, indicating that the failure was caused by a strain. Furthermore, when a person with presbyopia rests the eyes by closing them, or palming, he always becomes able, for a few moments at least, to read the fine print at six inches, again indicating that his previous failure was due, not to any fault of the eyes but to a strain to see. When the strain is permanently relieved, the presbyopia is permanently cured, and this has happened, not in a few cases, but in many, and at all ages, up to sixty and seventy.

The idea that presbyopia is "a normal result of growing old" is responsible for much defective eyesight. When people who have reached the presbyopic age experience difficulty in reading, they are very likely to resort at once to glasses, either with or without professional advice. In some cases such persons may be actually presbyopics, in others the difficulty may be something temporary, which they would have thought little about if they had been younger, and which would have passed away if Nature had been left to herself. But once the glasses are adopted, in the great majority of cases they make the condition worse. The patient finds that the large print which he could read without difficulty before he got his glasses, can no longer be read without their aid. Sometimes the eyesight declines very rapidly and the patient changes his glasses to higher powers quite frequently till no more power to the glasses can be added and still the patient suffers from discomforts in reading; if the patient does not go on to cataract, glaucoma, or inflammation of the retina, he may consider himself fortunate. Only occasionally do the eyes refuse to submit to the artificial conditions imposed upon them; but in such cases they may keep up an astonishing struggle against them for large periods. A woman of seventy, who had worn glasses for twenty years, was still able to read fine print and had a good vision for the distance without them. She said, the glasses tired her eyes and blurred her vision, but that she had persisted in wearing them, in spite of a continual temptation to throw them off, because she had been told that it was necessary for her to do so.

TREATMENT: Presbyopia is cured just as any other error of refraction is cured by rest. But there is a great difference in the way patients respond to this treatment. Some are cured very quickly, even in as short a time as fifteen minutes; others are very slow; but as a rule, relief is obtained within a reasonable period and many may find it difficult to discard glasses especially in dim or artificial light. Sun treatment, palming, blinking on white lines are a great help in curing presbyopia. Central fixation practices have proved very beneficial. Alternate reading of the distant chart and the reading test type proves very helpful. While reading, imagine as if the letters are written in a dark black ink. Imagination of a black dot is an advantage. When a patient looks at the white spaces between the lines of an ordinary book type, he can read for hours and no fatigue, pain or discomfort is felt. When discomfort and pain in the eyes is felt while reading, it is because the patient is looking directly at the letters. Concentration on candle flame is very useful.

A case of presbyopia of twelve years standing, using glasses of plus 3.5 was cured in three days by the use of his imagination. He could hardly read No. 3 of Fundamental card, and all the letters of the chart seemed to be grey. I reminded him that the type was in printer's ink and that there was nothing blacker than printer's ink. I asked him if he had ever seen printer's ink. He replied that he had.

Did he remember how black it was? Yes. Did he believe that these letters were as black as the ink he remembered? He did, and then he read the letters.

In another case of long standing the cure was very quick. It was impossible for the patient to read the fine print, and when he tried to read it he suffered from pain, headache and discomfort. I asked him to imagine the white spaces between the lines to be perfectly white. As soon as he imagined the white spaces very white by the memory of white paint, he began to read the fine print quite rapidly.

CAUSES OF FAILURE

1. A very common cause of failure is to look at the black letters and to pay no attention to the white spaces between the lines. Sometimes the imagination of the white spaces may be improved sufficiently so that one begins to read fine print, and almost immediately the vision is lost, because of the great temptation to look at the letters.

2. The patient stops blinking.

3. When people imagine the white spaces or white line, they close their eyes for too short a time, and when they open them, they are very apt to keep them open too long a time. It is really remarkable how difficult it is for some people to close their eyes for part of a minute and then open them for just a second.

4. Some patients while imagining the white line or spaces, test their eyesight. Testing the sight causes strain which always lowers the vision.

5. After some of the tests, the patients ask questions or make statements which show that they pay no attention whatever to the direction for avoiding strain. Such patients are not benefited.

6. Many patients seem to be bewildered by all sorts of things they have heard about presbyopia.

7. Others have a bad habit of outlining their own plan of treatment.

CASE REPORTS

1. One highly educated gentleman of fifty-five years of age had worn glasses since the age of forty. His distant vision was normal 10/10 with each eye separately. Then I gave him the reading test type. He held it at arm's length and began to read up to No. 5; but when I asked him to bring it closer to twelve inches, he could read only No. 1 and 2 without glasses. I told him not to worry about the reading but to see only the white lines in between the lines of fine print by blinking. After finishing the white lines each time he read one line from above. After reading each line from above he shifted to the white lines of the fine print. The treatment lasted for about thirty-five minutes. Soon he became able to read No. 6 at one foot distance. Then by the help of sun treatment and palming, he read the fine print.

2. Another patient of about sixty years was wearing glasses of plus five. His sight was tested on the test card and he read 10/40 with each eye separately and he could not read any print of the reading test type without glasses from any distance. He complained of headache and the pain in the back of his eyes, especially while working. The power of the glasses was increasing rapidly and a stage came when his doctor advised him not to increase the power any more. Glasses did not help him in relieving the discomforts. First, I directed him to remove the glasses and taught him blinking. Then I asked him to sit comfortably in the chair and palm for half an hour. Palming proved very useful. There was no pain or headache.

Now I applied Resolvent 200 and placed him in the sun. He enjoyed the sun for fifteen minutes with closed eyelids. In the meantime, I focussed the strong light by the sun glass on the eyelids for a few minutes only. It was the winter season, so he did not feel any discomfort in the sun. Then he turned the back to the sun and palmed again continuously for fifteen minutes. I put a cushion under his elbows to rest them. After fifteen minutes, when he opened his eyes, he read No. 5 from one foot distance. He also noticed that when he stopped blinking and stared towards the black letters, the whole line of letters became blurred. The patient then left the office. After 2 months' time, he again came to consult me. I was surprised to see that he could read the fine print from ten inches, and was reading newspapers without glasses.

3. Late Dr. S. Sinha, Bar-at-Law, ex-Finance Member of the Bihar and Orissa Government, began to wear glasses at the age of forty-six. His age was now 68. During this period, he changed his glasses many times under the direction of the famous eye specialists of London. The doctor in London prescribed a higher number (plus four spherical with slight cylinder) than before for both the eyes for reading. Glasses (plus one with slight cylinder) were also prescribed for distance.

I tested his sight with the test card and found that the vision of each eye was impaired. His vision was 10/50 with each eye, but the right eye was better than the left. Then I gave him the reading test type to read at one foot distance. All he could read with each eye separately was number 2 of the reading test type. With both eyes, he could read number 4. With the right eye, the letters were clearer than with the left eye. Then I thoroughly examined him in a dark room with the ophthalmoscope and arrived at the conclusion that the case was a simple one of hypermetropia. The strain was greater in the left eye than in the right.

Now, the treatment began. The first thing that I demonstrated was blinking. It was very difficult for me to educate him in right blinking. Sometimes he practised the right blinking. The second thing to educate him in was to glance at the white spaces in between the letters and the words.

Immediately I changed the treatment and asked him to practise central fixation. He performed this beautifully and became able to know that the letter regarded was seen best.

Sun treatment and palming proved miraculous in his case. He did not like to practise other methods than sun treatment and palming. The vision began to improve rapidly both for the distance and the near point. On the fifth day, his vision was as follows:

Right eye=10/20, No. 8 of fundamental card.

Left eye=10/30, No. 5 of fundamental card.

The gratitude of Mr. Sinha was profound and he has since then proved a loyal friend to this treatment. Very recently, he wrote to me in his letter that he consulted the famous eye specialist of Patna who was of opinion that the right eye was normal and the left eye had cataract. Further, Mr. Sinha wrote that he could read the finest print of the reading test type at one foot distance without the aid of glasses, and the 10ft. line from 10 feet distance with his good eye. As he had to do much reading work, it was difficult for him to keep up the relaxation, so glasses of plus 2.5 were prescribed for reading. Cataract developed in the left eye because he neglected to practise with each eye separately.

4. A patient of fifty was using glasses of plus 1.5. Distant sight was good. He could read No. 4 of the fundamentals card at 12 inches without glasses. While reading, some letters appeared in the form of many like a penumbra. When he made the eye little open by squeezing the lids or looked through a small hole made in the hand or paper, he could read fine print clearly. He was under the impression that the defect in his eye, due to some change in the lens, was permanent and he put this question:

Q. Why do I see clearly through a small hole if the decline in vision is permanent at my age?

A. When you see through a small hole, the rays are centred. If you can improve the sensitiveness of macula lutea to that extent that it may not allow distortion of the rays, you will be able to read as clearly as through a hole. The sensitiveness of the macula lutea is improved by central fixation and palming.

Sun treatment was not a help in his case, but he used to take sun treatment in the morning for a few minutes. Frequent practices of central fixation enabled him to read photo print within a few months. At times, during his office work, he used to relax his eyes by looking at the sky or by reading a chart hung in his room at about fifteen feet.

EYE TROUBLES IN OLD AGE

A patient's statement

It is a general belief that presbyopia or old age sight is a normal result of growing old, so at the age of fortytwo when I experienced difficulty in reading, the natural impulse in me was to consult an eye specialist and get glasses. Since then I have been using glasses and at the age of sixty-four the number of my glasses was plus 3.5. Though I knew Dr. Agarwal very well, it never occured to me that I could do away with glasses. I had taken the doctor's advice as a verdict that nothing else could replace glasses.

For sometime I was feeling heavyness or headache or strain in the eyes specially after reading and a sort of veil appeared before the eyes which made the vision defective. This trouble acted as a source of inspiration to consult our friend Dr. Agarwal whose wonderful cures we sometimes read of in *Mother India*.

About a week back one morning I happened to be in his eye clinic at the SCHOOL FOR PERFECT EYE-SIGHT. My glasses and vision were checked.

"Will you like to discard your glasses and get new vision?", he asked.

"It will be a blessing, but will it really be possible to

discard glasses at this age?", I counter questioned.

"Leave these glasses with me for a week and undergo a short course of eye education and see the result," he advised.

Very gladly I consented to his advice and started the treatment. To my surprise the vision began to improve from the very first sitting, and in a week's treatment I was able to read very small print easily. Now my near vision is as good as my distant vision. Dr. Agarwal has assured me that there will be no cataract or any other trouble if I could devote a few minutes daily to eye exercises. Though I keep a small number pair of glasses in my pocket I hardly use them.

The process of treatment that I followed was first to apply *RESOLVENT* 200 and face the morning sun for a few minutes with the eyes closed, then after washing the eyes with eye lotion I practised palming. When I closed the eyes and covered them with my palms I could see that it was all perfect dark before my eyes like black velvet. Then I looked at the candle flame while counting one hundred respirations. The next process was to shift the sight in between the lines of small print with gentle blinking and at frequent intervals I read the Snellen Chart placed in dim light at fifteen feet distance. This process enabled me little by little to read the small print. And when I could read the small print, the ordinary book print automatically became easy and legible. It was a surprise to me when the small print could be read easily. Then Dr. Agarwal explained everything.

A letter or a word is a combination of black and white. When you look at the white instead of concentrating on the black the eye muscles are relaxed and the eye is able to accommodate in a normal way. If people arriving at forty years of age adopt this simple process of reading some small print daily in good light as well as in candle light, they will be able to maintain good eyesight throughout their life and they will be saved from cataract and glaucoma and other eye troubles of old age. According to the view of Dr. Agarwal presbyopia is the result of strain, hence preventable and curable.

How is it fine print becomes clear after looking at some distant object? Answering this question Dr. Agarwal said that the strain at the distant object elongates the eyeball so as to accommodate while reading. Such a practice is useful when one uses plus glasses."

An inmate of the Ashram.

CHAPTER XVIII

FLOATING SPECKS (MUSCÆ VOLITANTES)

MANY persons suffering from imperfect sight especially myopia complain of specks floating before the eyes; these are called in medical terms "muscæ volitantes" or "flying flies". They are usually dark or black but can be of any other colour also, and sometimes they appear like white bubbles. They move somewhat rapidly, usually in curved lines, before the eyes, and always appear to be just beyond the point of fixation of sight. If one tries to look at them directly, they seem to move a little farther away; hence their name is "flying flies". They may have any shape. They are annoying, and sometimes alarm the patient.

Usually floating specks appear at one time and disappear at another time, but they are often present while one looks towards a uniform white surface. Sometimes they appear when the eyes are closed. Even in extreme cases there are periods, short or long, when they are not seen with the eyes open.

The literature on the subject is full of speculations as to the origin of floating specks. Floating specks are supposed to be due to the presence of moving, floating opacities in the vitreous. They have been attributed to disturbances of the circulation, the digestion and the kidneys and are also supposed to be an evidence of incipient insanity.

IMPORTANT POINTS — As regards the view that the floating specks are due to the presence of floating vitreous opacities, errors of refraction and physical disturbances the following points are worth considering.

1. Though floating specks are present usually in high myopia, they are absent in many high myopic cases. On the other hand they may appear before the eyes of persons of fairly good vision or in cases of small errors of refrac-

tion. Hence an error of refraction is not the cause.

2. They may be present in some cases suffering from disturbances of circulation, digestion and the kidneys, but they are absent also in most cases suffering from such disturbances even in an aggravated state. Further, they are also present in persons who have no such disturbance and are quite healthy. These facts do not tally with the idea that the floating specks are due to physical disturbances in the system.

3. If the floating specks are due to floating vitreous opacities, then we can safely say that the trouble is an organic one and that the floating specks ought to be seen with the aid of an ophthalmoscope or retinoscope, and that the patient should be able to see them before the eyes when they are open. They should not be seen when the eyes are closed because the retina is sensitive only to light and floating specks can be seen only when the retina is functioning.

On the examinations with an ophthalmoscope or retinoscope, these floating opacities are not found and the vitreous is usually found to be quite clear. Moores Ball writes in his Modern Ophthalmology: "Muscæ volitantes* show no opacities to the ophthalmoscope. They are exceedingly annoying, and often remain in spite of the correction of refraction errors and attention to the general health." Moreover, the patient may see them with the eyes closed or in darkness, and may not see them at times when the eyes are open. These facts do not harmonise with the theory that the floating specks are due to the presence of floating vitreous opacities.

4. Suppose there is an opacity in the vitreous of one eye

* In 1894 A. H. Banson of Dublin, reported the case of a man, aged 62 years, with normal vision, whose right vitreous humour "was studded everywhere with small, smooth, fixed spheres of a light cream colour." (Transactions of the Ophthalmological Society of the United Kingdom, Vol. XIV 1894. p. 101.)

Regarding the presence of an animal parasite, in cysticercus, in the vitreous, Moores Ball writes, "In many instances the patient complains only of loss of vision." (Modern Ophthalmology) and the other eye is all right. The vitreous opacity will not be seen as a floating speck because the mind has the faculty of fusing the images of both the eyes. Even if the good eye is covered, the vitreous opacity will not be seen as a speck unless it is quite big, dense and in the centre of the vision because the mind has the natural tendency to ignore to see the opacities in the form of speck or specks, just as when there is an opacity on the cornea or on the lens or when the retina has a blind spot, the mind does not perceive a speck before the eye as a result of the opacity or the blind spot. It is why many patients suffering from incipient cataract, keratitis punctata, and central opacity cornea do not complain of speck or specks before the eye though the vision may be defective due to such organic changes.

THEN WHAT CAN BE THE CAUSE? The truth about the floating specks is that they are the result of a strain of the mind, and when the mind is disturbed for any reason, floating specks are likely to occur. This strain is different from that which causes errors of refraction. In all cases of floating specks it will be found that the central fixation is lost partially or completely. By central fixation I mean that the letter or part of the letter regarded is seen best. For example, there is a small letter E on the Snellen Test Card; when the top arm of E is regarded at ten feet or more, it is seen more distinct than the bottom arm of E, and when the bottom arm is regarded, it is seen clearer than the top arm.

As a matter of fact the specks are never seen except when the eyes and mind are under a strain, and they always disappear when the strain is relieved. If one can see a small letter on the Snellen Test Card at ten feet or more with central fixation and then remember it mentally by central fixation, the specks will immediately disappear or cease to move; but if one tries to remember two or more letters equally well at one time, they will reappear and move. The trouble of floating specks is wholly functional and not an organic one.

Persons who have a fairly good vision and see floating specks also suffer from a strain. They do not possess good vision all the time. Their central fixation is frequently disturbed by seeing unfamiliar objects, wrong use of the eyes, worries, physical discomforts, lack of good sleep, etc. Floating specks may be present before one eye and not before the other, because there are two separate eyes, each functioning separately, one may strain and the other not. All relaxation methods are helpful in relieving the strain.

Patients who usually see floating specks while looking at a white wall or white clouds suffer from strain. Most people who did not see floating specks before, can see floating specks when they look at the sun, or any uniformly bright surface, like a sheet of white paper upon which the sun is shining. This is because most people strain when they look at surfaces of this kind.

The floating specks are present in cases of disturbances of digestion, heart and kidneys because these diseases cause strain on the mind and if the eyes and mind strain in such a way as to cause the presence of floating specks they will appear, otherwise not.

Patients who are benefited by correction of an error of refraction or by the treatment of the general system are those in whom the strain which makes one see floating specks is somehow relieved along with the correction of errors of refraction or the treatment of the general system.

Why a patient suffering from floating specks is declared to be suffering from vitreous opacities? There are several possibilities:

1. If the opacity is actually present in the vitreous, it will not be seen as a speck unless the opacity is dense and big enough in front of the central vision. The patient in whom there is the presence of the vitreous opacity usually suffers from floating specks as well. It is a mistake to conclude from this that floating specks are due to the vitreous

opacity.

2. Opacities in the vitreous may not be found but the doctor explains to the patient that the floating specks are due to the presence of vitreous opacities. It is only for the satisfaction of the patient.

3. Declaration of the presence of vitreous opacity may be due to the fact of the doctor himself suffering from this trouble and hence he sees it in the patient's eye or his mind is already hypnotised by the opinion of great authorities.

TREATMENT: Usually the strain that causes floating specks is easily relieved. Most cases suffering from floating specks have been benefited by the relief of strain with the aid of central fixation exercises. Some cases were cured in a very short time, a day or a week, while others took longer time. Seldom there were cases which took a very long time, a year or more, for the partial or complete cure.

In the treatment of floating specks it is very important at first to convince the patient that the trouble of floating specks is merely functional and that there is nothing wrong organically in the eye. The patient is warned not to try with his eyes whether he can see floating specks and is advised to ignore their presence altogether, putting no importance on their presence. Correction of the errors of refraction with or without glasses and the treatment of physical discomforts help in relieving the strain.

CASE REPORT

Many people with defective vision derive benefit from the use of glasses and also applied surgery when found to be necessary. Nevertheless there are also many with visual defects who are informed by doctors and specialists that nothing can be done for their complaint. In such cases some give up in despair and feel themselves doomed to a life of gradual deteriorating vision. There are however others who feel that somehow, somewhere there must be some one who could be able to help them and in their absolute faith invariably find that some one. This is found to be the case at the School of Perfect Eyesight, in Pondicherry where many "so-called" incurable eye defects have been rectified and if not completely cured, certainly improvements have occurred. One aspect which has been discovered is that such cases respond very well to the many varied exercises of relaxation perfected in the treatment given at the School. It reveals that the faith and the resolve not despair is an asset and assistance in the process of treatment.

Teachings dating from hundred years have stamped the consciousness of our Ophthalmologists so hard that they cannot conceive that the visual defects and floating specks could be cured partially or completely. A lady patient was suffering from floating specks of various colours all the time which often caused nausea and severe headache especially while reading. When the images appeared multiple, she experienced terrible mental strain. Her glasses improved the vision to normal to see distant objects but did not give any relief to floating specks. When she got disgusted with the prescriptions of eminent eye specialists and got no relief, she heard about the School for Perfect Eyesight. However, she wasted no time and one morning she was waiting with her parents to consult me. After a thorough check up I assured her that she would be all right and the improvement will be evident within a few days. These floating specks were imaginary, an imperfect expression of the mind due to mental strain and eye strain.

At first she was taught blinking to break the constant habit of staring. Often she played with the ball, practised long swing, moved the sight on the white lines of fine print and did long palming. Along with this set of exercises she was advised two things:

1. Ignore the presence of floating specks.
2. Do not experiment whether they are present or not.
By following this programme of treatment the feeling of

relaxation developed in her eyes and nerves of the head, also the floating specks were reduced considerably.

To tackle the problem more successfully she was taught central fixation and was given a picture card of Taj Mahal. At first glance the view-card appeared to be a flat coloured picture but by looking at it in a particular way without effort or strain she was able to enjoy it. The Taj appeared in all its glory in a bright light. The effect of the sun could be seen on the building, the shadows could be seen behind the persons walking in front of Taj. The three-dimensional effect could be produced easily with each eye separately. When she read Reading test type or the Snellen Eye Chart after viewing the picture, the letters appeared very dark; neither there was any floating speck, nor multiple images. The vision was quite normal without any complication. But as soon as she looked at objects with strain and made an effort to see them, the trouble recurred. So she was convinced that the cause of her trouble was the wrong habit of looking at things. By frequent practice of relaxation methods and by educating the eyes to function without effort, she got relief from her troubles. Then she enjoyed reading books and small prints. She was convinced that preservation of good eyesight was almost impossible without eye education.

Persons suffering from floating specks can be successfully treated by eye education and the art of seeing view-cards and pictures because the cause of floating specks is a strain. By doing so some have been cured in fifteen minutes, some in a month or so. Rarely there was a failure due to continuous habit of staring to look at the specks. In some cases the obscure part of the patient cherishes the presence of floating specks and recalls them again and again when they are not present. It becomes very difficult to treat such cases.

It is important to note that the patients suffering from floating specks and multiple images are usually

intellectuals. Due to long standing mental strain their memory
becomes dull and they usually forget their previous condition
when the improvement follows. They should be advised to
write their report daily. Due to obstinate old habit of
straining when the trouble recurs, they get depressed; and
the doctor ought to be careful that the depression of the
patient does not affect his consciousness.

CHAPTER XIX

SQUINT

Since we have two eyes, it is obvious that in the act of sight two pictures must be formed; and in order that these two pictures shall be fused into one by the mind, it is necessary that there shall be a perfect harmony of action between the two organs of vision. In looking at a distant object the two visual axes must be parallel, and in looking at an object at a less distance than infinity, which for practical purposes is less than twenty feet, they must converge to exactly the same degree. The absence of this harmony of action is known as "Squint" or "Strabismus" and is one of the most distressing of eye defects, not only because of the lowering of vision involved, but because of the want of symmetry in the most expressive feature of the face, which results from it, and has a most unpleasant effect upon the personal appearance.

DIVERGENT SQUINT: Eye turns out.

CONVERGENT SQUINT: Eye turns in.

VERTICAL SQUINT: Eye may look too high or too low.

ALTERNATING SQUINT: When the above conditions change from one eye to another, and sometimes the character of the squint changes in the same eye.

Sometimes the patient is conscious of seeing two images of the object regarded, and sometimes he is not. Usually there is a lowering of vision in the deviating eye which may not be improved by glasses, and for which no apparent or sufficient cause has been found. This condition is known as amblyopia. It is very common, and more prevalent among children than adults.

CAUSE: There are many theories about squint described in the text-books. They seem to fit in some cases but leave others unexplained, and all the methods of treatment are admitted to be very uncertain in their results.

The idea that the squint is due to a lack of harmony in the strength of the eye muscles that turn the eyes to various directions seems such a natural one that this theory was almost universally accepted at one time. Operations based upon it once were in great vogue; but today they are advised by most authorities only as a last resort.

The true cause of squint is a mental strain. Internal squint is produced by a different strain from the one which turns the eyes out, upward or downward. Double vision is produced by a mental strain different from that which lowers the vision or causes fatigue, pain or dizziness. Normal eyes have been taught to produce consciously all kinds of squint at will. This requires an effort which is variable in its intensity.

The fact suggests that since squint in all its manifestations can be produced at will, it should be considered curable by eye education. It is a well-known fact that many persons, including children, can learn how to produce squint and become able to relieve permanently all the varied symptoms of squint.

TREATMENT — The success of operative treatment is uncertain. Even if the operation is successful in correcting the squint, the sight of the squinting eye is not improved.

Glasses, though appear to do good sometimes, fail in many cases even to prevent the squint from becoming worse.

Fortunately squinting eyes often become straight spontaneously, regardless of what is or is not done to them. The fact is that squint is a functional trouble, originating entirely in the mind. It can be produced in normal eyes by a strain to see, and can be immediately relieved when the patient looks at a blank surface and remembers something perfectly. A permanent cure is a mere matter of making this temporary relaxation permanent. Permanent relaxation can be obtained by palming, swinging, central fixation, memory and imagination exercises. Imagination of a perfectly black dot or an object or a letter creates a sufficient mental control and hastens the cure of all sorts of squints.

TREATMENT OF YOUNG CHILDREN — 1. Children of six years, or younger, can usually be cured of squint by the use of atropine, a one per cent solution being used into one or both eyes twice a day for many months, a year, or longer. The atropine makes it more difficult for the child to see, and makes the sunlight disagreeable. In order to overcome this handicap, it has to practise relaxation, and relaxation cures the squint.

2. Mothers or nurses should cover the eyes of the babies while feeding them with milk, because the babies move their eyes in the opposite direction to the movement of their heads. For example, when they lie to the left, they move their eyes to the right in order to see something. They should be given milk from both the sides for it causes equal balancing of the eyes.

3. Children having no squint should be kept apart from children or other persons who have squint.

4. Sway the babies in a regular and gentle swing from side to side.

5. The cradle is a good help.

6. The game of hide and seek is a very interesting game for children and can be enjoyed for long periods with great benefit.

7. Swinging the body in a circular direction (like dancing) hastens the cure. Or the child may be held strongly enough by an adult to lift his feet from the floor and then swing the child in a circular way, and at the same time, the child is encouraged to look upward as much as possible. The little patients always seem to enjoy this form of exercise.

8. Games of all kinds have been practised with much benefit to the squint in children. Different games have been described in the cure of amblyopia.

9. Teaching the children with squint the names of the

different colours at a near or greater distance is of benefit. In the beginning, the size of the colours may need to be large to help the memory, imagination or sight. As the sight improves, the child becomes able to distinguish the colours of very small objects. One may need to spend half an hour or longer daily for some weeks in order to improve the vision for colours to the maximum.

10. Using the poor eye with squint for a period of time each day while the good eye is covered with an eye shade is of benefit to the poor eye and lessens the squint.

Children do not like to wear a patch, because no one likes to have the good eye covered for a length of time. At first the patch would be worn for five minutes each day and then the time gradually increased until the patient is able to wear the patch all day long.

11. Numbers and letters of the alphabet can also be taught to the child who has squint. Then every morning and evening the test card should be read with both eyes together and then with the poor eye alone, having the good eye covered with the palm or the patch.

12. Blinking and palming prove very efficient. If the child cannot palm himself, the mother may put her hand or the child's hands on the eyes and then talk about pleasant things with the child.

13. Cases of squint should be kept under the supervision of one who has a good sight. No one with imperfect sight ought to try to help such cases at home because it cannot be done successfully. The unconscious strain which is evident when the sight is not perfect always produces more strain in the squint cases which are under treatment.

14. Swinging and palming to be combined in a swinging game in which two children join hands and swing with music. Children should look at the ceiling while they swing. At times they disconnect their hands, stop the swing, and palm. Beneficial for all the pupils.

15. Game with splints. Keep the E or 'pot-hook' eye card

hanging in the room. Have the children sit at a table 10 or 15 feet from this eye card, and facing it. Request children to make a picture with splints of the fourth line or any other line of characters on the card. When reading this E card the child may indicate which way each 'E' points, by the splint or by finger.

FOR GROWN UP CHILDREN AND OTHERS

1. Blinking and Palming are very helpful in each case.

2. *Eye-shade* — Some patients are benefited by wearing a patch over the good eye, so that the patient is compelled to use the squinting eye for vision.

3. *Swinging* — Almost all cases of squint are benefited by the swinging practice. They can be taught to imagine, while the good eye is covered, that stationary objects are moving. In cases where the swing of stationary objects is not readily accomplished, any of the following methods may be effective:

(a) The forefinger is held about six inches in front of the face, and a short distance to one side. By looking straight ahead and moving the head from side to side, the finger appears to move. This movement of the finger is greater than the movement of objects at the distance but, by practice, patients become able to imagine not only the finger to be moving, but also distant objects as well.

(b) The patient may stand about two feet from and towards one side of a table on which an open book is placed. When he steps one or two paces forward, the book and the table appear to move backward. When he takes two or more steps backward the table and the book appear to move forward.

(c) The patient stands in front of a window and looks at the distant objects. By swinging the body from side to side, the window and its bars may be imagined to be moving from side to side in the opposite direction to the movement of the body, and the more distant objects appear to move in the same direction in which he moves his head and eyes.

(d) The patient stands ten feet or less from the Snellen Test Card and looks to the right side of the room, five feet or more from the card. When he looks to the right, the card is always to the left of where he is looking. When he looks to the left side of the room the card is to the right of where he is looking. By alternately looking from one side of the card to the other, the patient becomes able to imagine that when he looks to the right everything in the room moves to the left. When he looks to the left, everything in the room appears to move to the right. After some practice, he becomes able to imagine that the card is moving in the opposite direction to the movement of the eyes. This movement can be shortened by shortening the movement of the eyes from side to side.

4. Practice of central fixation with a familiar card, or a card whose letters are remembered, is one of the best methods known for curing the imperfect sight of squint and the squint itself.

5. Some patients of squint see best where they are not looking. To cure this condition (eccentric fixation) central fixation practices should be practised. The patient is told to look at the first letter on the line of the Snellen Test Card at some distance, and to note that the letters towards the right end of the line are blurred or not seen at all. By alternately shifting from the begining of the line to the end of the line and back again, the vision is usually improved, because eccentric fixation is lessened by this practice. Sometimes, it is necessary for the instructor to stand behind the card and watch the eyes of the patient. The instructor directs the

patient to look down when he sees that the patient is looking too far up.

6. To cultivate the fusion sense, training on stereoscope or amblyoscope will be helpful.

7. If the usual treatment of squint fails, it is well to teach such cases to see double. In many cases of squint the patient sees double images. These cases are more readily cured. This suggests that the persons who have squint may be taught how to produce double vision.

TREATMENT OF SQUINT BY WAY OF DOUBLE VISION

When the right eye turns in towards the nose and the left eye is straight, the letter or other object seen by the left or normal eye, is seen straight ahead, while the image seen by the right or squinting eye is suppressed by an effort and is not seen at all. To teach the patient to see with both eyes at the same time requires much time and patience. When double vision is obtained, the image seen by the right eye is to the right, while image seen by the left eye is to the left. We say that the images are seen on the same side as the eye which sees them. With the eyes closed, the patient is taught to imagine a letter, an object or a light to be double, each thing is imagined to be on the same side as the eye with which the patient imagines he sees it. With an effort, two images may be made to separate to any desired extent. By repeatedly imagining the double images with the eyes closed, the patient becomes able, with the eyes open, to imagine the double images to be separated a few inches or less, a foot apart or further.

With the help of the imagination of an object, palming, swinging and central fixation, the two images may be made to approach each other and merge into one; the convergent squint is thus cured temporarily. By a frequent practice the patient gets more control and is benefited more permanently.

Some patients of convergent squint have been cured by

teaching them how to produce a divergent squint. When the image seen by the right eye is to the left of the other image, it is called *crossed diplopia,* and with few exceptions a divergent squint is present. With the eyes closed a person with internal squint may become able to imagine the images crossed, in other words, he may become able to produce a divergent squint with the aid of his imagination. By repeated practices in this way internal or convergent squint is cured.

A *divergent squint* usually causes crossed diplopia. It is well to practise the production and the control of the crossed images. When this is done, the crossed images may be imagined to approach each other and form one. In some cases the imagination of the images to the same side is very helpful. Looking at the tip of the nose or a point of the pencil held at the nose produces convergent squint and thus this practice is helpful in divergent squint.

One can produce all forms of vertical, internal or external squint, and this process helps in the cure of squint. Direct the patient to close the eyes and place the fingers lightly on the outside of the closed eyelids. With the help of the imagination of the candle images one can move the right eye in, while the left eye remains straight and *vice versa.* The right eye imagines the image to be on the left while the left eye imagines the image to be on the same side. The patient can produce every imaginable form of squint with the eyes closed better than with the eyes open. With the eyes open, later, one becomes able to produce a squint in flashes or temporarily and then more continuously. It is interesting to tell by the sense of touch whether the eye was looking in, out, down, up or straight.

AN INTERESTING CASE OF SQUINT

Among the numerous patients we receive in the Clinic, myopic patients are many. Cases of squint are fewer. Patients who have been treated for this trouble have been usually children whose ages ranged from two years to twelve years. There are just as many cases of squint among boys as there are among girls, but those who have come to me for treatment were mostly girls.

An interesting person who caught my attention was a man of twenty-eight years of age. He had a convergent squint in both eyes, well marked in the right eye. When he looked in front, the right eye turned towards the nose so much that the black part of the eyeball touched the inner corner of the eye, while the left eye remained straight. This want of symmetry of both the eyes called squint had a very unpleasant effect as it made him self-conscious.

This patient had very good and symmetrical eyes up to the age of twenty-five but had acquired slightly a convergent squint in the right eye when he was in Switzerland, where he had suffered from chronic conjunctivitis. He had developed the habit of screwing his eyes to protect them from glare and smoke. The squint gradually increased and when the patient landed in India it was well marked in the right eye. A marked wrinkle had formed between the eyebrows, and it seemed from the expression of his face that he was frowning.

The patient consulted a prominent eye specialist who suggested two alternatives:

(1) An operation which is now seldom advised, and is admitted to be a gamble. According to the specialist it cannot be effectively performed in India and has slender chances of a success in any circumstances.

(2) Dr. Agarwal's methods of treatment which according to that specialist, were frequently, though not always successful.

The specialist had suggested to him to wear glasses of plus 0.5 which according to him would prevent the squint from worsening though they would not cure it. The patient never wore glasses.

The patient had practised some eye exercises as advocated by some physical culturists. He kept the head straight and moved the eye balls in various directions. Such eye exercises worsened the squint as they created more strain.

This patient visited my clinic to have a regular course of treatment. I found that his left eye had a normal vision and the vision of the right eye was a little below normal. When he looked at a letter of the Snellen Test Card with the right eye, the letter was not seen more distinctly than the other letters which were visible while fixing the sight on that particular letter. This indicated that central fixation was very defective in the right eye. Loss of Central Fixation in the right eye was an indication that the mind was under a strain and was experiencing difficulty in fusing the two images of an object received from the right eye and left eye separately.

CAUSE: The patient firmly believed that his squint was due to weakening of some of the eye muscles which turned the eyeball in various directions. When I told him that squint was produced by purely mental strain which was quite different from the type of strain which lowered the vision or caused pain and fatigue he was surprised and did not believe me at first. I explained to him that the trouble was purely mental and the squint was the physical expression of the mental strain.

There are two eyes and obviously two pictures are formed, one in each eye, but these two pictures are fused into one by the mind. This subtle fusion sense of the mind needs perfect harmony of action between the two eyes. In seeing distant objects the axes of the two eyes must be parallel, and in seeing objects at less than twenty feet the axes must converge to exactly the same degree. The absence of harmony in action of both the eyes due to lack of this fusion faculty causes squints.

Relief of a mental strain produces fusion faculty. If a person having a squint can remember an object or a dot perfectly while facing a blank surface the squint disappears completely. This indicates that the trouble of a squint is a functional defect and is relieved as soon as the mental strain involved is relieved either spontaneously or by rest and relaxation of the eyes. As the specialists believe this defect to be a purely physical one, and treat only the effect and not the cause, the trouble generally continues to exist in spite of successful operations and glasses. Even if the squint is corrected by an operation the vision is not improved and the necessary fusion does not take place. Normal eyes have been taught to produce consciously all kinds of squint at will. This requires an effort which is variable in its intensity. My son has perfect eyes, and can produce a convergent squint while trying to look at the tip of the nose and then can immediately relieve it but he feels great strain and experiences a lowering of vision when he does so.

These facts suggest that the squint is a functional trouble, originating entirely in the mind, and since squint in all its manifestations can be produced at will, it should be considered curable by eye education.

TREATMENT: Since squints are always caused by an effort or a strain to see, mental relaxation is a fundamental part of the successful treatment. The first thing that I said to the patient was to keep the upper eyelids down so that the eyes may express as if they were half open eyes. While keeping the upper eyelids down the patient learns gentle blinking. At times he squeezed the lids, and this was undesirable. He frequently threw a ball upwards or sideways and in following its movements he moved his head without raising the lids. I made him learn the art of relaxing the eyes by palming and swinging. He felt his eyes somewhat relaxed and the squint appeared less but he was very impatient to have a quick cure.

One of the best ways of curing a squint is to learn how to increase the squint or how to produce other kinds of squint voluntarily. This patient did not like such ways.

In the cure of squints it is necessary to obtain the best possible vision in each eye. As the left eye was already normal, the immediate purpose was to improve the vision of the squinting eye with a view to developing that fusion faculty which had been lost. Here, three types of exercises proved most beneficial.

1. USE OF AN EYE SHIELD OVER THE GOOD EYE. An eye shield was worn continually to enforce the functioning of the amblyopic or the squinting eye. This enabled the defective eye to develop central fixation.

2. CENTRAL FIXATION. By Central Fixation I mean seeing best where one is looking. The smaller the part of a letter regarded in this way, the better is the Central Fixation. Central Fixation is perfect when the eye is able to regard a small part of a letter of the twenty feet line of the Snellen Test Card at 20 feet distance.

A Snellen Eye Testing Chart was placed before the patient at a distance where his vision was very good, and this distance was five feet. When he looked just below the letter 'C' on the white back-ground, the whole letter was visible without any attempt to see it, but the bottom part of the 'C' appeared more distinct than the top part of the 'C'. In the same way when he shifted his sight to the top part it appeared more distinct. It took a second to shift the sight from the bottom to the top and then from the top to the bottom. Similarly he practised on smaller letters up to the twenty feet line. At times he closed the eyes and recalled the memory of black or white colour or an object. Then he increased the distance of the Snellen Test Card to ten feet, fifteen feet and twenty feet.

Practice of Central Fixation educated the eye to focus correctly. The result was that the vision of the defective eye improved so much that he could read the fifteen feet line at twenty feet. At twenty feet a small letter appeared as black as the big letter. When he slowly shifted his sight from side to side of a letter, the letter appeared to move from side to side with a pendulum-like motion.

3. USE OF MENTAL IMAGINATION. When the imagination is perfect the mind is always perfectly relaxed and the sight is quickly improved. With closed eyes the patient would imagine some object or person connected with his past, until he saw it vividly in his mind's eye. Then he would open the eye slightly and continue to imagine visually that object or person.

The memory and the imagination of a small black dot or a comma proved best because it could be retained in the memory easily for a longer time. When the dot was imagined perfectly, it was not stationary but moved in various directions with a slow, short, easy swing. An effort to remember it always blurred the picture of the dot and impaired the vision and a strain was immediately felt in the mind and the eye. When a dot was remembered or imagined perfectly, Central Fixation was manifest and the small letters of the chart at twenty feet were very dark and distinct, the eyes and the muscles of the face were completely relaxed. The strain which was caused by the contortions of the muscles of his eyes and face disappeared. There was a sense of calm well-being which was inseparable from the true relaxation of the eyes. The eyes became quite straight showing no trace of squint. Now the patient realized what eye strain meant.

Quite frequently the patient lost central fixation and relaxation, with the result that the squint appeared or the image of the right eye was suppressed and it appeared from the expression of his eyes that the right eye was not looking at an object.

Gradually the periods of relaxation increased so much that the flow of relaxation was continuous for hours together. The immediate relief to the eye from strain and squint and the consequent improvement of the vision were then quite remarkable.

Due to straining two teachers had developed divergent

squint in the right eye and it was a very annoying phenomena. They were quite all right by practising palming, long
swing and reading fine print in good light and candle light
alternately. They had learnt the right blinking.

A German lady used to get double vision and squint
while reading due to wrong use of the eyes. She kept the
head fixed and read without blinking. When she was asked
to shift the sight with the movement of the head and eyes
and to blink frequently while reading she became all right
in a couple of weeks. Often she went to the dark room
and read fine print in candle light with frequent gentle
blinking.

In another case the squint was almost cured by operation.

CHAPTER XX

DOUBLE VISION

When the eye regards two images of one object, it is called double vision or diplopia.

Homonymous Diplopia: When the image seen by the right eye is to the right of the image seen by the left eye.

Crossed Diplopia: When the image seen by the right eye is to the left of the other image. Generally, a divergent squint is present in such cases.

Cause: Eye strain, which is a mental phenomenon, is capable of producing in the eyes two images (diplopia), or many images (polyopia). The strain which causes a double vision is different from other strains. Even normal eyes, if taught to produce a double vision, can produce a double vision. This suggests that the strain is the cause of the double vision and relaxation is its cure.

HOW TO PRODUCE DOUBLE VISION

1. If one will press the lower lid of the eye with the forefinger, while both eyes are open, one can immediately produce two objects where there is only one. The harder the pressure against the lower lid, the further away the one object moves from the other. One is real and the other is, of course, an illusion. It is a good practice to do consciously where one is troubled with double vision. When a double vision becomes worse consciously, one is very likely to become able to cure this defect sooner than is usually expected. One can imagine how the patient must have strained his eye in order to produce the double vision constantly, not only while the patient was at work but at all times while he was awake.

2. Imagine two lights, one directly above the other, at

an angle of 90 degrees. When the strain will be sufficient the two lights would be seen on the vertical plane. With the help of the strain, the two images can be seen at an angle of 45 degrees, 60 degrees or 75 degrees. In short, one can produce double images close together or double images farther apart and at any angle.

3. To produce double images, one above the other, look at a light about ten feet away and strain to see a small letter just below it at an angle of 90 degrees.

4. Look above a light, or a letter, and then try to see it as well as when directly regarded. If the strain is strong enough, you can produce not only double images but an illusion of several lights, or letters (polyopia), arranged vertically. If the strain is still great enough, there may be as many as a dozen of them. By looking to the side of the light or letter, or looking away obliquely at any angle, the images can be made to arrange themselves horizontally or obliquely at any angle.

5. Most patients can see or imagine double vision by practising with a lighted candle or other object. When one is practising with a candle at twenty feet, two candles can be imagined five feet apart or one foot apart. If the objects are on the same level, they can usually be controlled much better than when one is higher than the other. In a case of convergent squint, it is quite easy to imagine the two objects as they should be imagined; the image of the right eye should be to the right, the image of the left eye should be to the left. When the two images are on separate levels, it is well to practise so as to attain the two images on the same level. This makes it easier to control the two images in other directions.

By alternately regarding the images without an effort or a strain, they will approach each other until they touch, overlap or become fused into one object. Then more practice should be done with the object of obtaining control of the location. By particular forms of effort the image of the right eye may be forced to the right. This should be practised for half an hour or longer, forcing the images seen by each eye to approach crossed. At first, the images are not controlled, they may cross and separate a wide distance, three feet or even six feet.

Treatment — 1. Blinking is a good help, because generally one or the other eye remains fixed.

2. Imagination of stationary objects to be moving is very important. Long swing practised with both eyes open, and then with the good eye covered is very helpful.

3. Patients should be educated how to see objects. One should drift the sight from one point to another of the object and imagine that to be moving in the opposite direction.

4. Palming practised several times a day.

5. Other relaxation methods may also be tried with benefit.

6. The good eye may be kept covered with an eyeshade for some time.

7. If the patient does not improve, educate him how to produce a double vision consciously and make the condition worse.

8. If the patient sees the letters double while reading, educate him the correct way of reading and writing.

9. In cases of squint, treat the squint.

CASE REPORTS

1. A patient while returning from Europe, suffered from a double vision. When he reached India, the trouble increased. He consulted different eye specialists in India. The doctors thought that the double vision might be due to paresis of external eye muscles; and that the paresis might be due to some toxin in the body. They reported the vision to be normal. They gave twenty-seven injections in the arm for the cure of the double vision, but the disease became worse. I examined him very thoroughly. The vision was normal, but I marked that at certain time, the eye changed into a

different shape and became blind. To know whether the double vision was due to a strain or not, I asked him to shift his eyes from one side to the other and blink while seeing any object. I placed my fountain pen before him. Now he shifted his sight from the top to the bottom and from the bottom to the top, and noticed that the pen jumped up and down. I asked him whether he saw the pen double. He said, "No".

"Now stop blinking and stare towards the pen," I said. "It is double now", he replied.

On certain other things, I demonstrated the fact that the cause of a double vision was simply staring. He agreed with my view and knew it perfectly that the cause of the disease was simply the wrong use of the eyes and not the paresis of the muscles. Shifting and swinging, sun treatment and palming helped him very much. In a week's time he became much better. Later, I received a letter from him that he had improved still more and now rarely got a double vision.

2. Many persons complain that they see two moons or more; and when they look at some objects for sufficient time, it becomes double and pain is felt in the eyes and head. Generally, the cause of this trouble is that people stare at objects with the upper eyelids raised, and do not blink at all. I have demonstrated this fact in several cases. Recently, a patient consulted me about double vision. He used to keep his upper eyelids raised all the time. Blinking was altogether absent. I taught him to keep the upper eyelids lowered always and blink frequently. I put the Snellen chart before him at 15 feet distance and asked him to look at C by raising the upper eyelids and by lowering the upper eyelids. Soon, he reported that the letter became double when he raised the upper eyelids but became single when he lowered the upper eyelids. He learned soon the secret of his cure, followed it sincerely and no more trouble remained in his eyes.

DOUBLE AND MULTIPLE IMAGES

A Case Report

Most Ophthalmologists do not believe that visual defects could be corrected by eye education and mental relaxation and they fit each patient with imperfect sight with glasses which are not indicated. Even to children of two to four years they prescribe glasses. Some such patients actually suffer from hypermetropia with its disagreeable symptoms of pain, discomfort and headache in reading. These cases when examined under atropine strain in such a peculiar way that the eyes become temporarily myopic with astigmatism. Prescription of minus glasses in such cases creates all sorts of disagreeable eye troubles as double vision, multiple images, floating specks, etc., and there is a rapid deterioration in eyesight. As their eye trouble increases more and more they go from one doctor to another in despair. Ultimately they get disgusted at the difference of their opinion about the diagnosis and treatment without any relief.

A college student had good eyesight but was afraid of examinations and hard studies in bright light, developed a strain in his eyes and began to read slowly, thus began to suffer from headaches, pain and irritation in the eyes. When he found double vision developing, he consulted one eminent eye specialist of his own town who examined him under atropine and prescribed minus glasses. By the constant use of glasses the strain in the eyes increased greatly, he found his eyeballs and the face muscles under some tension. Later on multiple images of bright objects began to appear and he experienced terrible strain in the head and eyes. It became almost impossible for him to read for more than a few minutes. His eyesight greatly deteriorated, even with glasses his vision was quite poor both at a distance and also near. By the continuous strain on the mind his memory became dull and he lost the charm of life. This patient was greatly puzzled when one eminent eye specialist diagnosed conical cornea and prescribed contact lenses which greatly increased the trouble. Then when he consulted another renowned eye specialist, the doctor found the cornea, the lens and all the other parts of the eye quite normal but could not help in any way to relieve the discomforts.

Seeing multiple images of an object is an illusion of imperfect sight caused by a strain of the mind, and when the mind is disturbed for any reason, it can add all sorts of imperfections for seeing clearly. By looking above a light with a staring look, and then trying to see it as well as when directly regarded, one can produce an illusion of two lights or more lights. If the strain is too great, there may be as many as a dozen images. By looking to the side of the light, the images will be seen horizontally.

Vision is a process of mental interpretation of retinal images. In other words our vision is our mind's imagination. Look at the white centre of letter 'O', the white centre appears whiter to the normal eye. But when the vision is imperfect, the imagination is also imperfect, the white centre does not appear whiter at different distances. Then if the strain is great, the mind adds imperfections to the imperfect retinal images. It is a great relief to patients to learn that these multiple images or other appearances are imaginary, and it helps them to bring the imagination under control. As it is impossible to imagine perfectly without perfect relaxation, any improvement in the interpretation of the retinal images means an improvement in the conditions which have led to multiple images or to a distortion of those images.

The first thing advised in this case was to discard the glasses so that the eyes may learn to blink and break the habit of staring. When rest is obtained by proper blinking, the vision is much improved and the discomforts disappear. When the eye discontinues to blink, it usually stares and tries to see. Blinking is beneficial when practised in the right way. What is the right way? Blinking when done properly is slow, short and easy.

Every morning the patient enjoyed sun treatment and practised palming for 10-15 minutes and did long swing. Often he educated his eyes to shift with the help of a ball which he moved from hand to hand and followed its movements. Shifting the sight on the white lines of small print without any attempt to read greatly helped the ability to read without any discomfort. By this process the left eye considerably improved but the right eye was not responding. Still it could hardly read Fundamental No. 1 and that too with shades and multiple images. So now the patient was advised to cover the left eye with an eye shield and develop central fixation in the right eye. When the right eye was able to develop central fixation, it began to read the Fundamental chart and in about two weeks was able to read the smallest print. By doing so the ability to read with both eyes greatly increased and one day this patient read forty pages at a stretch without any discomfort. He got convinced that reading fine print daily in good light and candle light is extremely beneficial to prevent and cure most of the discomforts of the eyes.

CHAPTER XXI

BLINDNESS OR AMBLYOPIA

When the sight is poor and cannot be improved promptly by glasses, the cause is usually due to amblyopia. The word amblyopia means blindness. In amblyopia the vision is less in the region of the centre of sight, and the part of an object or a letter regarded by an amblyopic eye does not appear best.

Some cases of amblyopia cannot count fingers. The vision in some cases is affected slightly or more. The field of vision is usually contracted. Sometimes the black letters regarded at three feet may seem to be brown or to have a tint of green or some other colour. The perception of colours varies greatly at different distances. In some persons the vision is quite good at one time while at other times the patient gets attacks of amblyopia. Amblyopia is usually present in squinting eyes.

The cause of amblyopia is staring. A patient had an attack of a temporary blindness. He was told that the cause of sudden attack of blindness was an eye strain. The eye strain was treated by the usual methods of relaxation very successfully. At one time he reported that if he took the trouble to practise relaxation methods he had no attack of blindness.

Dr. Bates mentions a very interesting case.

"A well-known surgeon suffered from attacks of blindness at regular periods. The blindness was complete so that he had no perception of light. The attacks of blindness worried him very much because he was afraid, while performing an important or dangerous surgical operation, that in the midst of it, would come an attack of sudden blindness which would tend to interfere seriously with his work.

The neurologists whom the surgeon consulted all told

him that he was threatened with insanity and that unless he took a long rest he might unexpectedly find himself blind and insane. Every ophthalmologist whom he consulted gave him a different pair of glasses to wear, none of which gave him any relief. He not only suffered from attacks of blindness but he was also bothered by illusions of sight.

He said nothing about the amblyopia at his first visit, but told me that he called on me to have something done for his eyes. He had many symptoms of discomfort and he would be very much obliged to me if I would cure him. While examining his eyes with the ophthalmoscope and seeking to find some treatment which would improve his vision, I discovered that he was suffering from amblyopia. Then he was told that the reason that his sight failed and that he had attacks of double vision was because of this amblyopia. Then began a great battle. The doctor knew a great deal about physiological optics and would not encourage me to treat him until he was convinced that I was right and he was wrong.

When he was in his office he said that where he knew there was only one light, he saw two, three, or four lights. The images in some cases were arranged one above the other and the distances between them varied within very wide limits. He said, however, that the principal illusion he suffered from was that it seemed to him that his hands and feet were double, sometimes more than double. The size of the double images varied; sometimes one image was four or five times as large as the other. In some cases the double images were arranged one above the other, while in other cases they were arranged in an oblique direction. When he looked at a Snellen Test Card hanging up in my office, the bottom lines were double and the colour of each line of letters appeared different. With the aid of central fixation this illusion disappeared and did not return.

To satisfy the surgeon I made repeated examinations of his eyes with the aid of the ophthalmoscope and each time

I reported that his eyes were all right and that there was nothing in either of his eyes which could explain the illusions from which he suffered. They did not come from any malformation of the interior of the eyeball but were imagined. He was very much impressed when I told him how to produce illusions of sight consciously whenever he so desired. He discovered that it was necessary to strain in order to do this and knowing the cause of his trouble made it easier for him to relieve it by doing away with the strain.

This doctor went through the World War and when he returned he came to my office and thanked me for what I had done for him. He said that he had not had a single attack of temporary blindness from the stare or strain of amblyopia, because knowing the cause of his trouble he was able to prevent it."

(2) Brijmohan was blind with his left eye. Although he was immediately taken to eye specialists of various places, he could not be cured, and the case was left as hopeless.

With the test card, the vision of his right eye was 10/200, but the left eye had only light perception. This is a copy of his prescription for glasses, which he had worn:

R. E. plus 1.0   L. E. plus 1.0

I examined him with the ophthalmoscope and found the eye in a normal state. The trouble was simply amblyopia in the left eye. While the examination was in progress, Brijoo's uncle was sorry because he was told by the doctors that Brijoo would always have to wear glasses to save the right eye; that nothing more could be done for the left eye. After the examination was over, his uncle exclaimed breathlessly: "Is not there any hope at all Doctor, please? Oh, say there is." I did not promise anything. I study each case that comes to me and help as much as I can. I explained the method of palming. By palming is meant to close the eyes and cover them with palms of the hands and shut out all the light; then to think of something. When I asked Brijmohan what he remembered while palming, he said, "I can remember very well the black beard of my teacher." At once a roar of laughter came out from all present at that time.

After palming for five minutes, with left eye he became able to see the big letter of the chart, but as soon as the letter began to become dim, he closed and covered his eyes. By repetition, he could see the big letter at one foot distance on that day and left the hospital with a smile. It was a matter of great joy for me also, because a ray of hope appeared in a hopeless case. Two days later, the boy came again and with him came his uncle, eager to hear more of the miracle that happened to Brijoo. The same practice was continued. The vision jumped from 1/200 to 2/200 in the left eye.

On May 13th, the fifth day, Brijoo came with his grandfather, who was anxious about him. His grandfather stood by the side of his grandson and beamed with happiness as he saw his little boy's sight improved. He was thankful to see the rapid progress in Brijoo's sight. This day, after an hour's practice, there was a wonderful change in his sight. The vision was 20/200 in left eye and 20/20 in right eye. Both went away smiling.

The sixth day was the last day of Brijoo's visit. He was anxious to go home. This day his vision became 20/60 in the left eye and 20/20 in the right eye.

After one month, I saw Brijoo again. Vision was 20/30 after palming and he could read fine print.

(3) Another boy was blind with the right eye. He came to know of this blindness at the time of the medical examination of his eyes in his school. I sat by his side and asked him to practise palming. His power of imagination was perfect. Whatever he imagined, he explained perfectly. He began to improve and after two hours' practice, he read the twenty feet line from twenty feet; and the fine print at nine inches distance. Such cases are very rare who respond to the treatment so quickly.

(4) Later, two boys came for treatment from Dehra Dun. Both of them had no vision in one eye. Simply palming did not help much. Sun treatment, swinging and palming proved very beneficial in these cases. After about two months, they could read and write very well and had no difficulty in seeing distant objects with the blind eye.

(5) Prasanna Kumar, aged ten years, was medically examined by the Health Officer and was found to have a slightly weak eyesight. He was put under an eye specialist who after examining him under atropine prescribed glasses of plus 0.5, but the use of glasses made the condition worse. Frequent eye examinations under atropine increased the strain and the boy became more or less blind.

I tested his sight, which was 3/60 or 10/200 for the distance and J6 for reading. The ophthalmoscope and retinoscope revealed everything to be normal. I explained to the boy's father that the blindness was simply functional due to a strain and that he would gain his normal sight within a short time by the relaxation exercises.

The boy was taught first the correct position of the upper eyelids and blinking. Every morning, he practised sun treatment and palming. I brought the Snellen Test Card near him, and pointed to the letter 'O' and asked him if he could imagine the letter with the eyes closed.

"Yes, I can imagine the letter 'O'," he said.

"All right," I said, "Imagine as if 'O' is moving away from you, and as it moves, it becomes smaller and smaller."

"Yes, it moves and it is a tiny 'O' at fifteen feet. Now, it comes towards me and becomes bigger and bigger," he replied.

Next day, he could keep up the memory of the tiny 'O' while looking at different objects. Then, he imagined the tiny 'O' on the top of each letter of the chart. Then, I asked the boy to shift his sight from side to side on the background of each letter, and imagine the small 'O' on each side of each letter.

"Yes, I am able to imagine the small 'O' while looking on each side of the letter on the chart, but I note one thing quite new. When I imagine 'O' to the right of the letter, the letter seems to me to be moving to the left and *vice versa*," he said.

Perfect imagination of 'O' and of a cricket game proved very beneficial in his case. On the fourteenth day, his sight became normal both for the distance and the near point. His father took the boy to the same specialist who had examined him before and found the boy having a normal sight.

(6) BLIND BABY — A baby of six months showed an attitude of indifference to his parents when they looked at him. His did not gaze at the toys or candle light. The father, assuming that his eyes may be defective, took him to many doctors who declared the baby to be congenitally blind. The father happened to see my small pamphlet "Psycho-Solar Treatment for the Eye" and got some hope of recovery. He got the baby admitted in my hospital.

First, I got the baby treated for indigestion by some homeopathic doctor and then the following treatment was tried:

1. Sun treatment as given to the babies.
2. Swinging the baby in the cradle having a toy tied at the top of the cradle. Certain types of toys, which made some sound, were placed by his side.
3. In the night time, the candle was lighted in front of his eyes, or the baby was moved from side to side before one or two candle lights.

After a few days, the child began to show signs of improvement and, after twenty days, he began to behave as a normal baby.

CHAPTER XXII

CATARACT

The opacity of the lens or cataract is caused by a strain in most of the cases. It is easy to cure or prevent it in the early stage. Some cases can be benefited in the advanced stage also if the degenerative changes have not taken place.

The treatment which brings about a persistent and durable relaxation always cures the cataract, but after a considerable treatment which may require several months or longer. There are a great many methods of treatment for bringing about a relaxation needed in the cure of the cataract. The measures employed are not injurious; in fact, there is no possibility of making the condition of the eye worse. I do believe in operation when necessary, when medical treatment fails to cure the trouble. The operation should only be performed when other measures fail because after all the operation is never free from a danger.

It is well to emphasise the fact that the same method of treatment to obtain a relaxation is not beneficial in all cases.

1. REST: Closing the eyes and resting them, or covering the closed eyelids with the palm of one or both hands without exerting any pressure on the eyelids, has improved many patients. Palming for five minutes hourly is usually beneficial. With the eyes closed and covered, it is well that the patient allows his thoughts to drift from one thing to another without trying to remember one thing in particular all the time. By thinking of pleasant things, it is often possible for the patient to forget that he has eyes and in this way a large amount of relaxation is obtained. Many people with cataract, when they close their eyes, feel that they are doing what they were told and cannot understand why they obtain very little benefit. Closing the eyes is not always followed by a relaxation and rest. In short, there are many

patients with cataract who strain their eyes more when they are closed than when they are open. These patients are directed to practise the universal swing, the long swing, and the variable swing.

2. SWINGING: Swinging is very helpful in the cure of the patients standing or sitting. Some patients have practised the swing while sitting in a chair for many hours during the day. When tired, they would alternate with palming. When the swinging is done correctly, it is restful and a benefit not only to the cataract, but to other conditions of the eye. By practising the swinging exercises, many patients soon become able to imagine stationary objects to be moving in the opposite direction to the movement of the head and eyes. A great benefit derived from the sway is that the stare, the strain and concentration are prevented. Babies with cataract are benefited when the mothers sway them in their arms.

3. MEMORY AND IMAGINATION: Perfect memory is a great help in the cure of cataract. When the patient remembers some letter as well with the eyes open as with the eyes closed, the vision is improved, and the cataract disappears.

When the patient stares, concentrates or makes an effort to see, the memory and the imagination always become worse. Patients who cannot control the functions of the mind are difficult to treat. The patient himself and others can feel with the tips of their fingers lightly touching the closed upper eyelids that the eyeball becomes harder when an imperfect sight is remembered. But when a perfect sight is remembered, the eyeball becomes as soft as is the case in the normal eye. Patients with a perfect memory, consciously or unconsciously, remember letters, colours and other objects continuously, without any strain or fatigue. These cases are favourable and recover from the cataract.

4. FINE PRINT: Some patients acquire the ability to read without glasses very fine print held a few inches from the face. When such patients are recommended to read the

fine print many times daily, the cataract becomes less and the vision improves.

5. Concentration on candle flame while counting 100 respirations and reading fine print in good light and candle light prove very beneficial.

6. SUN TREATMENT: Patients with cataract seem to improve more decidedly from the light treatment than from any other kinds of treatment. Congenital cataract or cataract present from birth, is benefited and often cured in the same way. Cataract produced by an injury to the eye has improved and occasionally been cured by sun treatment. So often the light treatment benefited many kinds of cataract that the use of the light has been strongly recommended in all cases.

When taking the sun treatment, it is best to let the eyes become accustomed to the sun by mild treatment at first. Have the patient sit in a chair with his eyes closed and his face turned towards the sun. He should slowly move his head a short distance from side to side. The movement of the head prevents concentration of the sun's rays on one part of the eye. After some days of the treatment, or when the patient becomes more accustomed to the light, one may use the sun-glass with added benefit. Direct the patient to look down and while he does this, lift the upper eyelid gently, exposing to view the sclera or white part of the eye. Now, with the aid of the sun-glass, focus the sunlight on the forehead or the cheek, and then rapidly pass the concentrated light over various parts of the sclera. This requires less than a minute of time. It is not good to be in a hurry. One should wait until the patient becomes sufficiently accustomed to the sun to permit the upper eyelid to be raised while he looks down, exposing the sclera only. It is important that the patient be cautioned not to look directly at the sun.

Sun treatment, palming and reading of fine print daily have proved very beneficial in the prevention of cataract.

A patient of fifty had early cataract and high myopia. Sun treatment and central fixation exercises were a great help in curing his cataract and in the improvement of his sight.

SENILE CATARACT: A patient had cataracts in both the eyes — more in the right. The famous eye specialists of Delhi advised him to have the right eye operated, and to wait for the left eye for about a year. The patient was afraid of the operation. He came to me to have my opinion. After a thorough examination, I found that the degenerative changes had not taken place in either eye. I said to him; "The left eye will become able to read the finest print and see distant objects well, but the right eye will improve so much as to avoid the necessity of operation." At the beginning of the treatment he could only perceive the movement of the fingers with the right eye, and with the left eye, he could read No. 4 of the Reading Test Type. In the beginning of the treatment, the imagination of the white line helped him much. Later on, sun treatment and palming proved very efficacious. He was taught the ways of reading and writing. His vision improved. He could read the finest type of the Reading Test Type with the left eye and the seventh line 2 Q C O G D E C of the Snellen Test Card C, pocket size, with the right eye. The patient continued the treatment.

SECONDARY CATARACT: A poor old man came to the hospital for cataract operation in the right eye. He had mature cataract, which was removed on the second day. Unfortunately, a small part of the covering of the lens called capsule, remained inside the eye. The eye was bandaged. On the seventh day the wound healed up, the bandage was removed, but the patient could not see anything. The whole pupil was white. The patient felt very sorry. I asked him to come again after two months for another operation. At the same time, I gave him one medicine to be dropped into the eye after taking sun treatment twice daily, morning and evening. After one month, he returned. He could see everything. The whole pupil was perfectly black. He needed no operation. I was surprised to see the wonderful cure of nature. I asked him what he had done. He said, "I used to sit in the sun for one hour in the morning and for one hour in the evening, with closed eyes, and used to move my head and body from side to side as you said. Then I used to come to a cool place and drop the medicine that you gave. For seven days, there was no improvement in the vision, but after that, the vision improved little by little. I began to enjoy the sun for an hour and a half each time."

Another patient having a secondary cataract was treated on the same lines. That case also was benefited and required no operation.

BLACK CATARACT: A young man of about 32 years was blind in the left eye. He came to the clinic. This was a case tried by many doctors. I examined him in the dark room thoroughly under atropine with the ophthalmoscope. The pupil was quite dark and gave no red reflex. This was a case of black cataract in the left eye. He suffered from no other disease like diabetes or kidney troubles.

I had no hope of his recovery without operation and I explained everything to him clearly; the patient had great faith in me. He induced me to prescribe some medicine for him. On his request, I gave him one phial of Resolvent A, to be used after taking sun treatment both morning and evening. After one month, the patient returned again and said, "Doctor, I am very grateful to you. Your medicine acted like a magic. I can now read and write big letters. This medicine is finished, kindly give me one phial more."

I took out his ticket and was simply surprised to know that a case of black cataract was giving me such gratifying report. I examined him again and found that the pupil was not black now and gave a red reflex. Then I tested the vision. He could read 10/80.

The patient continued the treatment for some time more. The whole cataract had dissolved and his blind eye began once more to work very well.

CATARACT AND EYE EDUCATION

A Patient's Statement

"What is cataract? The doctor said, "The eye just like a camera, has a transparent lens. When somehow the lens shows signs of opacity in its substance then this condition is called cataract."

It was a shock and a matter of great anxiety to me when the doctors at Madras diagnosed early cataract in my eyes and asked me to wait for an operation till the cataract was matured. Though after the operation cataract patients usually become all right yet sometimes the patient suffers much after the operation and in some cases the vision is lost. However, I did not like the idea of an operation and in a depressed state returned to Pondicherry. Next day I consulted Dr. Agarwal in his eye clinic; his reputation for curing eye troubles is prevalent in the Ashram. At first he put some questions regarding my eye trouble and physical fitness. My eyesight had started deteriorating by proof reading in light and the bright electric number of glasses was frequently increased. When I questioned why the number of glasses was increased so often, Dr. Agarwal said that due to strain in reading hypermetropia had developed.

Even with a high power of plus glasses my vision was gradually failing, the eyes tired quickly and the vision became hazy, headache and strain increased in reading. Then after a thorough examination in the dark room the Doctor said that this kind of cataract was due to strain, hence preventable and curable and there was nothing to worry about. If I could undergo his treatment faithfully for some months, the cataract would dissolve and the vision improve. I felt very happy and consented to take the treatment. For six months I was regularly attending the eye clinic and doing different eye exercises. I enjoyed the sun treatment and palming and I played with a tennis ball to practise football swing. In this exercise the ball is moved forward with the foot and as it rolled forward the ground appeared to move backward. This observation of apparent movement greatly helped my eyes to relax their muscles. And by doing this exercise in relaxation my physical health also improved. My diet was also regulated.

When I looked at the candle flame while counting 100 respirations I felt as if I had gone into a trance, there was peace in the head and in the nerves of the body. The eyes felt a sort of power in them. I knew Yogis used to concentrate on the candle flame and they maintained good eyesight.

For two months I had completely discarded glasses and allowed my eyes to accommodate themselves in different conditions of life. Then Dr. Agarwal advised me to use glasses of less power and practise with them the methods of eye education in reading. So daily I read small print with glasses in good light as well as in candle light. After six months I found that my eyesight had become normal with glasses and all the discomforts had been chased away. It became quite convenient to read and see proofs for hours. Now two years have passed and I maintain good eyesight and daily devote some time to eye exercises because preservation of good eyesight is impossible without eye education. When Dr. Agarwal re-examined my eyes in the dark room with his instrument, he found no trace of cataract. And such a good condition of eyes I shall maintain now by eye education."

A Patient

CHAPTER XXIII

GLAUCOMA

Glaucoma is a serious disease of the eyes which, some years ago, was considered incurable when chronic. In most cases, the eyeball is usually too hard and this is the symptom which, more than any other, is the strongest evidence we have to indicate to us that the affection in the eye is one of glaucoma. The field of vision is contracted on the nasal side and the pupil is usually more or less dilated. One characteristic symptom is the apparent appearance of colours around the flame of a candle or some other similar light.

Glaucoma is a disease of adult life and seldom occurs in children. Its uncertainty is unusual. For example, a person with normal eyes and normal sight may retire to bed perfectly comfortable. Sometime in the middle of the night, he may be awakened by a very intense pain, with a total permanent blindness in one or both eyes from glaucoma. In a limited number of cases, the pain may be absent, although the vision may be partially lowered. The sudden onset may not occur, but one or both eyes may slowly, without pain, after a long time, a year or longer, become totally blind.

The results of the various methods of treatment, which were suggested and practised, have been so disappointing, that we hesitate to foretell what may happen after any of them have been practised.

It is a very welcome discovery made by Dr. Bates that the relief of eye strain always lessens tension, relieves pain and improves the vision. The discovery that relaxation methods cured glaucoma suggested that the cause was due to an eye strain. Experimental work proved this to be true. All methods of treatment, which promote relaxation, always benefit glaucoma.

Absolute glaucoma is a serious disease and the state of

the patient can become so bad that a large amount of pain and a total blindness may be produced. The pain may be so severe that many ophthalmologists feel justified in removing the eyeball to bring relief. While many cases of absolute glaucoma obtained much relief from pain after the removal of the eyeball, there were too many cases which still had severe trouble, even after such an operation. A strain which produces the absolute glaucoma is really a mental strain and not a local one entirely.

Glaucoma may be produced solely by the memory of imperfect sight. If a person with normal eyes and normal vision presses lightly on the eyeballs through the closed eyelids and remembers or imagines a letter "O" with a grey, blurred outline very imperfectly the eyeball can be felt to increase in hardness. When the patient remembers a letter "O" perfectly, the hardness of the eyeball disappears and the eyes become normal as they were before. These experiments are offered as a proof that the memory of an imperfect sight is a strain which may produce glaucoma, and that the memory of a perfect sight is a relaxation, which will relieve glaucoma.

Some of the best methods of producing relaxations are the practice of the long swing, the universal swing, palming and sun treatment. There are some people who cannot practise a certain swing correctly until after weeks of instruction. They are full of excuses and are quite ready to find fault with the method rather than their own lack of practising it properly. The memory of letters and other objects seen by central fixation becomes very much better in a short time. Imagination of a thin white line or the white centre of the letter "O" whiter than the rest of the card is very helpful. Frequent enemas, fasting, dropping of lemon juice in the nose once or twice a week, and a regulation of diet have proved beneficial in glaucoma patients.

The following are the reports of cases who had come to me for treatment: —

1. A man, aged thirty-five, was all right when he went to bed. During the sleep, he got severe pain in the right eye. Redness increased and watering continued. The eyeball became very sensitive. The vision was lost. The doctor whom he had consulted before coming to me had said that he was suffering from glaucoma and iritis. The eyeball was hard. This sort of inflammation had taken place two or three times before also and every time the inflammation had continued for about two months.

The first thing that I did was that I gave him a strong enema which caused about ten or twelve motions and much mucus passed with the faeces. Then I gave a vapour bath to his face for a few minutes. Sun treatment and relaxation exercises were practised. The whole trouble subsided within twenty-four hours, the eyeball became soft, and the patient became all right in a week's time.

2. An old woman had been suffering from glaucoma without pain, the vision was 1/20. By the help of an enema, regulation of diet, sun treatment and palming, she began to read fine print of Hindi test type within a fortnight.

3. Another old lady was suffering from inflammatory glaucoma with severe pain in the temples. First a few drops of ginger powder mixed in milk were dropped in the nose, which brought out much discharge through the nose and mouth. This sort of treatment helped in relieving the pain. At bed time, the patient took a purgative which caused about four motions. Sun treatment and swinging exercises were practised. The redness subsided in a week's time and the vision began to improve. Since then, she did not get any attack of glaucoma.

4. An old man had absolute glaucoma and the vision was totally lost in the right eye and there was perception of light in the left eye. He had undergone an operation after which there was some vision in both the eyes; but the vision gradually went on diminishing. Such cases are incurable and no benefit is generally possible.

CHAPTER XXIV

EYE STRAINS

One strains in different ways and the ways of treating strains are different; but generally, the patients suffering from a simple eye strain are benefited by the right use of the eyes, sun treatment and reading of photoprint. In some cases, symptoms of eye strain are peculiar; and it seems as if the patient is suffering from granulations or trachoma, and the treatment of granulations does little or no good in such cases. Though relaxation exercises generally relieve the strain, yet, in certain cases, one feels a strain while practising them because the patient somehow is not able to relax. Many people have asked me for help in choosing the best method of treatment of their particular eye trouble. A woman, aged sixty, complained that she had never been free of pain; pain was very persistent in her eyes and head. She also had continuous pain in nearly all the nerves of the body. The long swing, she practised 100 times and it gave her great relief from pain. The relief was continuous without any relapse.

The long swing was practised by some other people with a satisfactory result. It seemed that the swing was indicated for pain. Later on, however, some patients attempting for a relief from pain were not benefited by the long swing. Evidently, one kind of treatment was not beneficial in every case. A man suffering from trigeminal neuralgia, which caused great agony in all parts of the head, was not relieved at all by the long swing. Palming seemed to be more successful in bringing about a relief. Furthermore, there were patients who did not obtain benefit after half an hour of palming; they however obtained complete relief after palming for several hours.

The experience obtained by the use of relaxation methods

in the cure of obstinate eye troubles has proved that what was good for one patient was not necessarily a benefit to other patients suffering from the same trouble and that various methods must be tried in each case in order to determine which is the most beneficial for each particular case.

(1) A lady patient had a slight but persistent redness in the eyes and a little swelling of her lid margins since childhood. It was not possible for her to come out even in ordinary light without the aid of dark glasses. She could not read without discomfort, though her eyesight was normal. For many years, she was treated for trachoma. Glasses increased the trouble. She was very doubtful if my treatment would help her at all.

Generally, patients having photophobia are greatly benefited by sun treatment, but it was unusual in her case that sun treatment helped her only a little. Blinking and swinging before window bars proved very beneficial, and within twenty days her eyes became perfectly all right.

(2) Another lady of a royal family suffered from redness in the eyes, usually after sleep and after seeing a cinema. It was painful for her to read a page or to write a letter. The doctors treated her for trachoma for a sufficiently long time. Her eyesight was normal. Sun treatment was a great benefit to her. She practised swinging and central fixation exercises for a few minutes every day after the sun treatment. She was educated in the right way of reading, writing and seeing the cinema. Within ten days, she became perfectly all right; and one day, when she went to the cinema and got no redness or strain, she was surprised to note the benefit.

(3) A woman, aged sixty, recently came to me for treatment. She had worn glasses for more than thirty years to improve her vision not only for the distance, but also for the reading. Bifocals made her eyes feel worse and produced a greater amount of discomfort than any other glasses. Three years ago, the vision of the right eye was

good and she could read a newspaper with her glasses. With the left eye, she could not read, even with glasses. Her vision for distant objects was imperfect and was not improved by glasses. Sometimes, the right eye had a good vision while the vision of the left eye was much less. On other occasions the vision of the left eye was good, while that of the right eye was very imperfect. She had been to see a great many eye specialists for treatment, but none had been able to fit her properly with glasses for the distance or for the reading. All these eye specialists admitted that they did not know the cause of her imperfect sight. She was fitted with many pairs of eye glasses, no two of which were alike. Some doctors prescribed eye drops, others internal medicines. With the hope of giving her relief from the agony of pain which she suffered, various serums were administered. Some eye specialists treated her for cataract, others for diseases of the retina, optic nerve and other parts of the interior of the eyeball.

She was suffering from eye strain or a mental strain, which produced many different kinds of errors of refraction. When she strained her eyes, she produced a malformation of the eyeballs which caused imperfect sight. This condition had been temporarily improved by glasses. In a few days or a week, however, the glasses had caused her great discomfort and made her sight worse.

I made a very careful ophthalmological examination, but found no disease in any part of the eye. Her eyes were normal, although the vision was imperfect. I emphasised the fact that if she wished to be cured permanently, it was necessary for her to discard her glasses and not to put them on again for any purpose. This she consented to do.

The use of her memory and imagination helped to improve her vision. She committed to memory the various letters of the Snellen test card with her eyes open, regarding each letter; her memory or imagination of the letters was good. When she closed her eyes, not only could she remember or imagine each letter perfectly black, but she also could remember the size of the letter, its location, its white centre and the white halos which surrounded it. With her eyes closed, she could remember the whiteness of the spaces between the lines much better than she could imagine it with her eyes open. With the aid of the retinoscope, I found that when she imagined with her eyes open, there was no myopia, hypermetropia, nor astigmatism present. When she suffered from pain, however, the shape of the eyeball was changed and her vision always became worse.

The patient demonstrated that the normal eye is always normal when the memory or imagination is good. When the memory or imagination is imperfect, the vision of the normal eye is always imperfect.

A Snellen test card with a large letter "C" at the top was placed about fifteen feet in front of her. To one side was placed another Snellen test card with a large letter "L" at the top. She was unable to distinguish the large letter "L" with either eye, but she could read all the letters on the "C" card, including the bottom line, with the aid of her memory and imagination. With a little encouragement, she became able to imagine the large "L" blacker than the large "C", although she could not distinguish the "L". In a few minutes, when she imagined the "L" blacker than the big "C", she became able to distinguish it. By the same methods, she became able with the help of her memory and imagination to imagine small letters on the large "L" card to be as black as the letters of the same size on the "C" card. By improving the blackness of the small letters on the large "L" card, and imagining them perfectly black alternately with her eyes open and closed, the small letters became visible and she was able to distinguish them.

When this patient looked fixedly at, or centred her vision upon, one part of a large letter at six inches, she found that it was difficult, and it required an effort, to keep her eyes open, and to look intently at one point. She also found that, by looking at other letters and trying to see them all at once, or by making an effort to see all the letters of one word simultaneously, her vision was lowered. When she was advised to look at the white spaces between the lines, she said that it was a rest and that the white spaces seemed whiter, and the black letters then seemed blacker. When she avoided looking directly at the letters, she became able to read some of the large print.

After she had imagined the white spaces between the lines to be whiter than they really were, it was possible for her to imagine the thin white line. This line is imagined along the bottom of a line of letters where the black of the letters meets the white of the white space. She was not always sure that she looked at the white spaces although she planned to do so. When she tried to read and felt pain or discomfort, she was unconsciously looking at the letters; but when she looked at the white spaces and succeeded in avoiding the letters, she felt no discomfort and she was able to read almost continuously without being conscious that she was looking at the letters. When she practised the relaxation methods and did not stare, nor tried to see, her vision became normal.

CHAPTER XXV

QUESTIONS AND ANSWERS

Q. 1. How is it that on some days I can read the Snellen Test Card up to the 15ft. line and on others only up to the 20 or 30ft. line?

A. When the eyestrain is less, the vision is always improved, continuous practice will make the sight perfect.

Q. 2. How can one overcome the stare if it is unconscious?

A. Keep the upper lids lowered and blink consciously. While walking, keep the sight on the ground and avoid seeing in the front at a long distance. Never look at an object for more than a few seconds at a time. Shift your gaze frequently.

Q. 3. When I wake up in the morning, I suffer from pain in the eyes and head. It becomes difficult for me to open the eyes and sometimes the eyelids are swollen. What remedies would you suggest to me for their relief?

A. Practise the long swing or run in a small circle before going to bed for 15 minutes; repeat the same soon after you wake up from the sleep. Some patients are benefited by muscular exercises which may produce sufficient muscular fatigue. Or when you go to bed lie comfortably on the back and let one hand lie on the chest, the other on the abdomen. Breathe just ordinarily without raising the chest. Take 100 or 200 breaths by raising and lowering the abdomen.

Q. 4. When I look towards an object even for a very short time, I see two images. The lines of letters become double when I begin to read. Will you please suggest some treatment for me?

A. Lowering the upper eyelids and blinking will prove very helpful. When you look towards any object imagine it to be jumping with your blinking. Learn the methods of improving the near sight and read photo print.

Q. 5. How long does it take to cure an average case of myopia?

A. Some patients are cured more quickly than the others. The length of time is uncertain, as patients differ in their response to treatment.

Q. 6. Why is my vision worse on a rainy or cloudy day than in broad daylight?

A. Because you strain to see on a dark day.

Q. 7. I am practising the methods to cure myopia and astigmatism. Sometimes, for short periods, I see perfectly, then things fade away. Can you explain this?

A. This is what we call getting flashes of a perfect sight. With a continued practice, these flashes will come more frequently and eventually will become permanent. Thus you will be cured.

Q. 8. In the case of an illness when one is unable to practise with the Snellen test card or stand up, what method is used?

A. Blink frequently and shift your eyes from one point to another. Turn your head slightly from side to side on the pillow or close your eyes and think of something pleasant.

Q. 9. I am short-sighted (myopic) and can read and write very easily without glasses; but my doctor has advised me to use glasses all the time. I can see all right at a distance but feel a strain in near work with glasses. What do you advise?

A. Myopic patients should not use glasses for near work as their reading sight is quite good.

Q. 10. I had good eyesight in my young age but somehow after sometime my distant sight became defective. The doctor prescribed for me glasses for constant use to check further deterioration in my eyesight. In spite of my constant use of the glasses and frequent consultations with the doctors, my eyesight went on decreasing. Finally the doctor advised me to discard reading and writing. What is your advice?

A. Your eyesight would not have deteriorated if the doctor would have given you three suggestions along with the use of glasses.

    a. No glasses for near work.

    b. Avoid strain by frequent blinking.

    c. Take sun treatment every morning or practise central fixation for 5 minutes.

Reading at a near point does not increase myopia, but always lessens it. Look at a card of fine print at six inches from your eyes and read it as well as you can. Now make an effort to see it better and note that your vision for the near point is lowered, while the ability to read the fine print at a greater distance is improved.

Q. 11. Being a high myopic patient I cannot see a short distance even with glasses. Reading also is difficult. You advise me to discard the glasses before beginning to practise. How can I pull on with the work and the treatment?

A. Take leave from your work for a month or so and improve your sight as much as you can. Then you may take the lowest power of the glasses. Use them only in case of a necessity. Avoid their use in reading and writing. Keep up your practices once a day at least.

If you are not able to take leave from your work or are unable to discard glasses, learn blinking and take sun treatment daily to check further deterioration.

Q. 12. My vision, after practice with the card, is good, but I cannot sustain it. What means can I use to have a continuously good vision?

A. Acquire a continuous habit of imagining stationary objects to be moving easily, until it becomes an unconscious habit. Make blinking and the position of the upper eyelids perfect.

Q. 13. I have improved my sight by palming, but when I read for any length of time, the pain returns. What do you advise me to do?

A. When you read and your eyes pain you, it means that you are straining your eyes. Frequent blinking, palming and reading photo print may help you.

Q. 14. What treatment helps most people?

A. Blinking, sun treatment and palming.

Q. 15. My eyesight is normal but when I read I get pain in the eyes and head. The doctor tried glasses but they increased the trouble. What should I do?

A. It is because you do not read with central fixation. Your eyes try to see many words at a time. Hold the book at a distance where you see the print best. Read fine print daily in dim light. Blink gently.

Q. 16. What causes redness and a smarting sensation of the eye, even when plenty of sun treatment has been given? Should one continue with the sun treatment under the circumstances?

A. Take the sun treatment frequently for five or ten minutes at a time daily, increasing the length of time until the eyes become accustomed to the sun. The eyes should always be benefited after the sun treatment, and one should always feel relaxed. When done properly, the redness and smarting should disappear soon. If the eyes are not benefited, it is an indication that you strain while taking the sun treatment. Alternate the sun treatment with palming or closing the eyes to rest them.

Q. 17. If I am reading in the sun I can see the print perfectly and my eyes do not trouble me, but if I raise my eyes and look at any other object, every thing seems blurred and there are coloured spots before my eyes. Is this caused by the sun or the manner in which I read?

A. The sun is beneficial to the eyes, but the glare of light on the white page produces a tension of the nerves. The sun treatment should help you. Practise it for ten to thirty minutes. When looking at objects do not raise the upper eyelids but raise the chin. Keep the upper eyelids lowered.

Q. 18. Are the dark sun glasses harmful?

A. Dark glasses are injurious to the eyes, but one may use a very light colour Crooks A only when there is much glare.

The eyes need the light of the sun. When the sun's rays are excluded from the eyes by dark glasses, the eyes become very sensitive to the sun when the glasses are removed. It is very beneficial to face the morning sun for ten to thirty minutes with the eyes closed.

Q. 19. If I am worried at night and lie awake, my eyes burn and pain, and I have a feeling that a magnet is drawing my eyes through my head. What causes this and what is the cure?

A. This is caused by a strain of the mind. Just before retiring and just after rising in the morning, practise the long swing.

Q. 20. My eyesight is normal both for the distance and for the reading. What should I do to keep them perfect?

A. Blink frequently. Take sun treatment for about five minutes daily in the morning. Read fine print at six inches distance with each eye daily.

Q. 21. What causes my vision to become blurred upon a sudden confusion or when I have a number of activities coming at once?

A. The fact that your vision becomes blurred at such times is a proof of your eccentric fixation. Do not try to see or do several things at once. Practise central fixation, seeing the part regarded best and other parts not so clearly, all day long.

Q. 22. It is very hard for me to think in terms of black and white. Is there some other method which is just as beneficial?

A. Yes, letting your mind drift from one pleasant memory to another will accomplish the same results.

Q. 23. Would the reading of fine print at four inches be

helpful?

A. The reading of fine print at four inches is usually helpful.

Q. 24. I have a normal vision, but after reading for a while, my eyes feel strained. Would you still consider I have a normal sight?

A. If your eyes feel strained you are not reading with a normal vision.

Q. 25. It is difficult for me to find time enough to gain a perfect relaxation. What would you suggest?

A. You have just as much time to relax as you have to strain. Practise relaxation all day long. Whenever you move your head or eyes, notice that stationary objects move in the direction opposite to the movement of your head or eyes. Walking about the room or on the street, the floor or pavement appears to come towards you, while objects on either side of you move in the direction opposite to the movement of your body. Remember to blink frequently just as the normal eye does. Constantly shift your sight from one point to another seeing the point regarded more clearly than all other parts. When talking with anyone do not stare. Look first at one eye and then the other, remembering to blink.

Q. 26. Can you explain why I see yellow and blue spots after looking at the sun?

A. You are straining. Do not look directly at the sun until your eyes are more accustomed to it. Practise sun treatment with the eyes closed.

Q. 27. Is working or reading under an electric light harmful?

A. It is not harmful to read in the electric light if the eyes are used properly and if there is not a dazzling light on the paper.

Q. 28. Why do some people see better by partly closing the eyes?

A. People with poor sight can see better by partly closing

the eyes, but when they have a perfect sight, partly closing the eyes makes it worse. This is a good test for the vision of ordinary objects.

Q. 29. Please explain what you mean when you say "imperfect sight, imperfect memory."

A. If you see an object imperfectly, blurred or grey instead of black, you cannot remember it perfectly. What is imperfectly seen is "imperfect sight." The memory of the imperfect sight of anything is "imperfect memory".

Q. 30. If test types can be seen more distinctly with the eyes partly closed, is it advisable to read that way?

A. No, it is not advisable to read that way because it is a strain, and alters the shape of the eyeball.

Q. 31. Can a patient while practising your method carry on his daily work as usual?

A. Yes, most patients continue their work just the same without the use of their glasses even though they find it difficult at the start.

Q. 32. Can the vision be improved after the lens has been removed for cataract?

A. Yes.

Q. 33. What causes styes?

A. Infection, which is always associated with eye strain.

Q. 34. Trying to make things move gives me a headache, palming gives me more relief. Why?

A. Making an effort to do a thing will not- help you. When you are walking on the street, the street should go in the opposite direction without effort on your part. Some people get more relief from palming, while swinging helps others more.

Q. 35. Should one imagine a thin white line along the top of a word or sentence or just at the bottom?

A. If you can imagine it at the top as easily as you can at the bottom do so, otherwise imagine it only at the bottom.

Q. 36. If strain is the cause of imperfect sight, why are

not all affected in the same way? Why is it that some have myopia, others astigmatism, etc.?

A. Different people react in different ways to a strain. Some have mind strain, some nerve strain, some physical strain, etc. All these tend to cause various ailments. One's temperament also has a great deal to do with it.

Q. 37. Is gazing on green grass turf or at the blue sky beneficial to the eye?

A. Yes, because there is nothing to stare at.

Q. 38. Is application of antimony for discharges and watering from the eyes, beneficial?

A. Yes.

Q. 39. Is *"Sirsasan"* i.e. standing on the head with feet above for a few minutes, which reverses the blood circulation, good for the eyes?

A. Yes, but one should learn it first with the help of a teacher. It is important to note that the eyes should remain closed while practising *"Sirsasan"*.

Q. 40. Is putting of rose water drops or honey beneficial to the eyes?

A. Yes, but not in every case.

Q. 41. Is occasional weeping beneficial in any way?

A. Yes, but weeping in the love of the Lord is highly beneficial.

Q. 42. By using glasses, why does the degree of myopia remain the same in some persons, and goes on increasing in many others, causing severe damage sometimes?

A. When the doctor prescribes glasses, he is not able to distinguish whether in a particular case myopia will increase. He prescribes glasses with the idea that the progress of myopia will be prevented. In some cases it does not increase because, somehow, the person begins to see the objects without effort; but in a majority of cases myopia goes on increasing because the habit of straining is not relieved.

Q. 43. How can one give rest to maintain at least the remaining vision when the eyesight is very defective? Is reading harmful?

A. The eyes are meant to see. Their right use should be learnt. Reading can be made a means of great benefit to the eyes, if one reads in the right way. Correct position of the upper eyelids, sun treatment, palming and swinging are helpful means to give rest to the eyes. Myopic patients strain more when they discard reading and keep on looking at distant objects. It is generally forgotten that myopia is caused by straining to see distant things and not near things.

Q. 44. How is it that you have prescribed different methods for the same disease? How can one know the right treatment for himself?

A. The main object in the treatment is to obtain a relaxation free from strain. Whatever method will relax the mind of the patient will be beneficial to him. If some method does not bring good results, it should be discarded and some other method should be tried; but in certain cases, practical demonstrations by an experienced man are absolutely necessary; because mistakes in the exercise are liable to be made. Moreover, intuition guides one to adopt particular lines of treatment.

Q. 45. It is said that rubbing the eyes after meals improves the eyesight. If it is so, then why particularly after meals?

A. It is right that rubbing the eyes after meals improves the sight and helps in relieving headache and other discomforts; but rubbing the eyes in the right way is useful and I call this method "Contact swing". Its practice is specially useful after meals because the blood circulation in the hands is increased and a sort of magnetism is developed. If one can improve the blood circulation in the hands at other times, the contact swing will have the same useful effect.

Contact Swing: Close the eyes and keep the palms of the hands on them. Now move your face up and down while the hands remain in position. You will feel that hands move down when you move your face up and *vice versa*. Practise for 5 minutes or more several times a day. It is very helpful after the meals. This contact swing relieves the strain, gives relaxation, and is very useful in headaches and defective vision.

Q. 46. Is it good to fix up the sight in between the eyebrows as is said by some persons?

A. It is useful if one can concentrate in between the eyebrows through the internal eye and if the external eyes act simply as an expression of the inner eye. It is harmful if one simply uses the external eyes to fix up in between the eyebrows.

Q. 47. If a person with imperfect sight has a good imagination, why is his sight imperfect?

A. One needs a perfect imagination at all times and in all places to have a perfect sight. Persons with imperfect sight, who have a good imagination, fail to use it; they suppress it and imagine things imperfectly by an effort which, of course, lowers their vision.

Q. 48. What precautions should I take at the time of the medical test of my eyes?

A. When you are called for the eye-examination, remember three points:

1. Cover one eye with the palm of the hand and not with the fingers. The finger causes pressure on the eyeball, and consequently the sight becomes defective. You are unable to read the smaller letters with that covered eye.

2. Keep the chin a little raised, and the upper eyelids lowered.

3. Blink gently on each letter.

Q. 49. Has looking at beautiful things and at the moon any good effect on eyesight?

A. Yes, it is soothing and useful no doubt; but one should take care not to stare.

Q. 50. What should be the distance to practise with the

Snellen Test Card?

A. The best distance to practise with the Snellen Test Card varies widely. Generally the patients begin to practise at ten feet distance and gradually increase it to twenty feet distance. If no improvement is manifest in a few minutes, it is well to try practising on one card at a near point where the vision is good and to FLASH the more distant card alternately.

Q. 51. Are eye troubles always due to some defect in the eye?

A. Not necessarily. Many a time eye troubles are not due to any defect in the eyes. Also normal vision is not a sure test of good eyes. The eyes are sensitive to many kinds of disturbances elsewhere in the body or mind. Hence, it is wrong to prescribe glasses immediately as soon as one complains of some defect in the vision. If the eyes are not seeing easily and correctly, there is a reason for it. Glasses can only relieve the effect but cannot touch the root of the trouble.

Q. 52. Why some people like to put on glasses even when they know the efficacy of natural methods?

A. Because people think that something may be done for them by some scientific means. They find it difficult to do anything by themselves, hence they like to put on glasses and see well. There are others who have an obstinate habit of using the eyes in a wrong way; they lack in perseverance and make half-hearted attempt, and are satisfied with partial or temporary improvement and prefer to put on spectacles. Some people believe strongly in the natural methods and fanatically discard glasses without taking proper care to eliminate the strain; this usually makes the condition worse and ultimately they are forced by circumstances to wear specs. There are others whose defect is high and are advised to use glasses also along with relaxation methods.

Q. 53. Why does the vision of persons having defective

vision vary without glasses when the degree of error of refraction may be the same or when a person having a higher degree óf myopia may see better than the other person having less degree of myopia?

A. The act of seeing depends mostly on the interpretation of the mind, and people differ in their habits and training to give better selective interpretation of the picture.

Q. 54. How does the act of seeing take place?

A. Seeing is a complex process depending on five factors — object of seeing, organ of sight, sense function, interpretation of mind and attention of inner mind. To see perfectly the eye should have full contact with the object to see. Then the external mind should be at rest so as to give correct interpretation. Then the inner mind should pay attention to see the object. When one is concentrated in painting or thinking, then many things may pass before the eyes but one may be unable to say what he saw or may give a vague idea.

The eye without the mind will mechanically photograph the image but will not interpret it. The mind without the eye can imagine the images previously seen, but will not tell you what you are seeing now. Correct seeing must be a perfectly coordinated action between mind and eye.

Q. 55. How the mind can be educated to coordinate properly with the eyes?

A. Generally people look at things but do not actually see them. They carry no impression, their minds are asleep even if their eyes are normal and open.

To improve this coordination of the mind with the eye, observe things intelligently as a woman observes another woman's dress. Close the eyes whenever possible.

Q. 56. What care should be taken in the case of a baby?

A. The newborn baby should be kept for a few days in a semi-dark room so that bright light may not affect the retina. At night a candle or a deepak may be burnt so that the baby may develop fixation of sight. Keep the baby in a cradle and in quiet and restful surroundings.

Q. 57. I am an artist. How the strain can be avoided in fine drawings?

A. It is not the fine drawing or any other such work which is the cause of strain, but rather the way in which it is done. Learn the correct use of the eyes and relax at times in between the work.

Q. 58. Can the cases of retinitis and chroiditis be benefited by your treatment?

A. There is a general belief that cases of retinitis and chroiditis or optic atrophy are due to some disease of the general system as syphilis, diabetes, focal sepsis etc. and treatment is given in the orthodox way, but the results are very discouraging. Good results follow by food reform and relieving constipation along with relaxation and visual training.

Q. 59. What do you suggest to prevent the formation of cataract?

A. Sun treatment, palming, reading fine print daily. Regulation of diet, sipping of considerable quantity of water to which a few drops of lemon may be added. Avoid such things which may clog the digestive system.

Q. 60. I practise several times a day and am able to improve the vision considerably but the improvement soon fades away after the practice. Why?

A. Exercises are useful and necessary to acquire the right habit, but it is the constant and correct use of the eyes which gives lasting results of improvement.

Q. 61. What is best to prevent cataract?

A. 1. Apply Resolvent 200 in the eyes.

2. Concentrate on a candle flame while counting 100 respirations.

3. Read fine print in good light and candle light with or without glasses.

Q. 62. I am presbyopic and use glasses of plus 2.5 for reading. When I go to a hill station, my eyesight is improved and I read the newspaper without glasses. Can you explain this fact?

A. Looking at the greens and seeing the things moving in the opposite direction while climbing up produces relaxation in the eye muscles, hence the sight is improved. Strain is the cause of your defective vision while relaxation is the proof of your improved vision.

Q. 63. Why do you recommend reading in dim light for a myopic patient?

A. Strain of reading in dim light causes hypermetropia, so it becomes helpful in myopic patients. After reading some small print in dim light for sufficient time with a little strain brings definite improvement in the distant vision of a myopic patient.

Q. 64. You recommend reading fine print in dim light and close to the eyes, these ideas are quite opposite to the orthodox belief. How do you justify your standpoint?

A. Those who advise you to read big print in good light at a long distance are your parents and teachers and doctors, they are mostly above forty, and at this age they lose the faculty of reading small print in dim light and at a near point. What suits them, they advise to others also. But for young and children reading fine print in candle light is extremely beneficial. You can test for yourself whether you read better in bright electric light or in candle light.

Q. 65. I am hypermetropic. What do you advise for me?

A. Place the Snellen Eye Testing Chart at 15 ft. distance in dim light. Hold the Fundamental chart to read in good light. Make an effort to read the distant chart, then shift your sight on the white lines of the Fundamentals with gentle blinking. Alternate. Strain at a distance will lessen the hypermetropia and finally make the eye normal.

A SPECIMEN OF TREATMENT CHART

Take the following treatment morning and evening: —

1. First apply the medicine Resolvent 200 with a rod in each eye.

2. After the application of the medicine sit facing the sun with the eyes closed for about 3 minutes. While taking the sun treatment, move the body gently from side to side like a pendulum.

3. After sun treatment come to the shade and wash the eyes with water and Ophthalmo.

4. Now sit comfortably with the eyes closed and covered with palms (palming) for about 5 minutes.

5. After palming, practise the following with both eyes and with each eye separately.

6. Swinging exercise for about 5 minutes.

7. Central Fixation on Om chart or Snellen Eye chart.

8. Read fine print or photographic type reduction with gentle blinking in good light and candle light alternately.

9. Read the Snellen Eye Chart at 10 feet without and with glasses. Blink gently at each letter.

10. Adopt correct habits of blinking, reading, writing, sewing, seeing cinema etc.

11. Drop Sollux in the eyes after meals and bed time and palm for 5 minutes.

HOW TO PROCEED WITH THE TREATMENT?

The normal eye has three illusions:

a. When the sight shifts from side to side of a letter, the letter appears to move in the opposite direction. This is swinging.

b. The letter regarded appears best. This is central fixation.

c. The white centre of a letter appears whiter. This is imagination.

These three illusions of the normal eye are reduced or are absent in the defective eye. So to improve the vision it is necessary to develop the normal illusions.

The defective eye loses the frequency of shifting and becomes more or less immobile. Therefore mobility is essential. In the first week develop mobility by blinking education, long and short swing, variable swing, circular swing, game of ball, table-tennis, walking and by observing the side objects moving in the opposite direction. By creating mobility all pain and discomfort and fatigue of the eye fades away, one feels relaxed.

The defective eye loses the faculty of central fixation. It tries to see a large area at a time and develops eccentric fixation. So to develop central fixation three main exercises are needed step by step:

a. Take the Snellen Eye Chart in hand, shift the sight on the line of letters, from one end to the other. By doing so the whole line appears to move in the opposite direction, and the letter regarded appears clearer than the other end letter of the chart.

b. Shift the sight from side to side of each letter, the letter appears to move in the opposite direction and the letter regarded in this way appears best.

c. Shift the sight from top to bottom of the letter and observe two things: when the sight shifts from top to bottom and bottom to top of the letter, the letter appears to move in the opposite direction and the part of the letter regarded appears best.

So in the second week develop the faculty of central fixation, read the booklet *Divine eye* in fine print several times a day in good light and candle light. Myopic patients should avoid using glasses especially in reading. Maintain relaxation by frequent palming and gentle blinking.

To the defective eye the white centre of the letter does not appear whiter than the margin at varying distances. So there is loss of imaginative faculty and the mind adds many other imperfections to the imperfect image received from the eye. So it is necessary to develop the faculty of interpretation of retinal images. This is achieved by imagination exercises. So in the third and fourth week improve the sight by imagination exercises.

a. Take the chart in hand and observe that the white centre of the letter 'O' and other letters appears whiter at a distance where the sight is best. Gradually increase the distance. Or take two charts — one in hand and the other at five feet distance. Look at the white centre at the near chart and then at the distance chart. Alternate.

b. Shift the sight on the white lines in between the lines of print in the Fundamental chart or fine print. When the sight shifts from side to side, the lines of print appear to move in the opposite direction.

c. Take view-cards and develop the art of seeing as described before in this book. The flatness of the picture will disappear and three-dimensional character of the picture will increase the beauty of the picture and the vision will be improved.

For myopic patients two important hints:

1. Avoid glasses in reading at least.
2. Read in dim light or candle light but not under bright electric light.

For presbyopic and hypermetropic patients two important

hints:

1. Avoid glasses for distance at least.

2. Keep the Snellen Eye Chart in dim light at about 15ft. and make an effort to read it. But hold the book in good light and make no effort to read. Reading Fine Print in good light and candle light alternately is extremely beneficial.

If the person remain constipated and there is mental tension, take an enema once a week. Regulate the diet.

If there is pain or discomfort, strain or headache or double vision in reading, it is an indication that the person tries to concentrate the sight on the black part and makes an effort to see consciously or unconsciously. Any sort of complaint in reading indicates wrong way of reading. This trouble can be easily tackled by the following process.

1. Application of Resolvent 200 or 500 in the eyes.

2. Sun treatment, eye wash and palming for 5 to 10 minutes.

3. Shift the sight on the white lines of Fundamental chart or Fine Print without trying to read it. When the shifting is perfect with gentle blinking, the lines of print appear to move in the opposite direction and the letters become more prominent. Continue till perfection is achieved.

4. See the view-cards and read *Divine eye* booklet several times a day in good light and candle light.

When the eyes become dull and lustreless, Tarpana Treatment is very helpful. For the Tarpana Treatment study the book *Secrets of Indian Medicine*.